Working with adults
at risk from harm

e the last date shown below.

Working with adults at risk from harm

Margaret Greenfields, Roger Dalrymple and Agnes Fanning

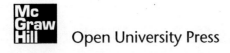

Open University Press

Open University Press
McGraw-Hill Education
McGraw-Hill House
Shoppenhangers Road
Maidenhead
Berkshire
England
SL6 2QL

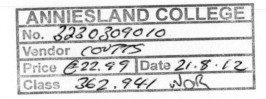
email: enquiries@openup.co.uk
world wide web: www.openup.co.uk

and Two Penn Plaza, New York, NY 10121-2289, USA

First published 2012

A catalogue record of this book is available from the British Library

ISBN-13: 978-0-33-524122-4 (pb) 978-0-33-524123-1 (hb)
ISBN-10: 0-33-524122-0 (pb) 0-33-524123-9 (hb)
eISBN: 978-0-33-524124-8

Library of Congress Cataloging-in-Publication Data
CIP data applied for

Typeset and ebook compilations by
RefineCatch Limited, Bungay, Suffolk
Printed in the UK by Ashford Colour Press Ltd., Gosport, Hampshire.

The *McGraw·Hill* Companies

Contents

Contributor biographies

Jill Aitken is a registered mental health nurse who has had a personal interest in the care of patients with epilepsy (particularly older adults) throughout her professional career. Her doctoral research was undertaken into the psycho-social impacts of the onset of epilepsy in later life.

David Bailey is Traveller and Diversity Manager for Fenland District Council where he specializes in equality and diversity activities and outcomes for the community. His career spans over 30 years in Local Government and he has previously worked for the Greater London Council, Lewisham Borough Council and Essex County Council in a wide range of senior positions. He advises many other Councils and, among his other activities at present, David is the Chair of Fenland Diverse Community Forum, Chair of the East of England MAF Chairs Forum, and a member of the Local Government Association Community Cohesion Task Force.

Jennifer Burton is Senior Lecturer in the Department of Social Work at Buckinghamshire New University, having worked previously as an operational manager for a range of community-based services for learning disabled adults. She is currently researching and co-writing a text on 'personalization' in social work provision.

Caroline Cole is London area manager for the Rehabilitation of Addicted Prisoners Trust (RAPT), a charity which helps people with drug and alcohol dependence move towards, achieve and maintain drug- and crime-free lives. For the past 15 years she has also been a freelance lecturer in higher education, working most recently at the universities of Oxford and Kent.

Roger Dalrymple is Reader in Education at Buckinghamshire New University. His research and publications explore the role of innovations in pedagogy and assessment in widening access to higher education.

Agnes Fanning is Principal Lecturer and Department Manager for Primary Care and Public Health at Buckinghamshire New University. Her research and publication interests are centred upon provision for the older person in a current of healthcare reform and demographic shifts.

Jo Edwards is Senior Lecturer and Practice Learning Coordinator in the Department of Social Work at Buckinghamshire New University. She has worked extensively with children with disabilities, within the child protection arena and also with adults with physical disabilities, specializing in those with drug and alcohol dependency issues.

Michael Farquharson is Senior Lecturer in Learning Disabilities at Buckinghamshire New University where he is Course Leader for the BSc (Hons) Epilepsy and the Advancing Care in Epilepsy (Post-qualifying Short Course). He is responsible for liaising with the National Society for Epilepsy to meet the training needs of their staff and specialist nursing professionals.

Margaret Greenfields is Reader in Social Policy at Buckinghamshire New University and Director of the University's institute for Diversity Research, Inclusivity, Community and Society (IDRICS). She has over 20 years' experience working with Gypsies, Travellers and other marginalized and excluded communities and has researched and published widely on the topic of social inclusion for nomadic people and regularly acts as a policy advisor with a variety of policy agencies and government departments, including the Equalities and Human Rights Commission, the Department for Communities and Local Government and national charities. Margaret is co-editor with Colin Clark of the best-selling *Here to Stay: The Gypsies and Travellers of Britain* (2006).

Lalage Harries is an integrative counsellor who has worked for the NHS undertaking brief, crisis and long-term counselling with diverse client groups. She has a particular interest in gender and sexuality in relation to mental health. Lalage is currently employed as Deputy Coordinator of Red Balloon Centre, an educational facility for vulnerable young people where she directs the centre's therapeutic programme.

Tennyson Mgutshini is currently Associate Professor in Mental Health Nursing at Indiana State University in the USA. He has over 12 years' experience working within mental health in the United Kingdom as a clinician, specialist community mental health practitioner, policy maker, service manager and as a lecturer in mental health. His work has focused particularly on marginalized groups within mental health. In particular, his PhD explored service user attributions for hospitalization with significant focus being placed on the unique vulnerabilities faced by the most severely ill.

Melanie Parris who is herself profoundly deaf and has a hearing dog, is Senior Lecturer and Practice Development Tutor Social Work at Buckinghamshire New University. She has worked with a range of service user groups, including older people, disabled adults and disabled children. She has also been employed as a community development worker, and a research associate at the University of Birmingham. Melanie's key professional interests are disability issues, service user involvement in social work education, and social work practice.

Kate Potter is Senior Lecturer at Buckinghamshire New University where she leads the Specialist Community Public Health Nursing PG Dip and BSc (Hons) Programme for Health Visitors and School Nurses. She has a special interest in child protection and safeguarding vulnerable individuals. Prior to taking up a role in higher education Kate worked as a health visitor for 13 years and has extensive experience with vulnerable families.

Acknowledgments

Grateful thanks to Melanie Havelock, who commissioned this volume, and Della Oliver and Katherine Hartle, who oversaw its completion; and to the editors' families.

Every effort has been made to trace and acknowledge ownership of copyright and to clear permission for material reproduced in this book. The publisher will be pleased to make suitable arrangements to clear permission with any copyright holders whom it has not been possible to contact.

Foreword

Mark R.D. Johnson
Professor of Diversity in Health and
Social Care, De Montfort University

In the 1960s, as a riposte or challenge to his perception of oversensitivity to difference (what we now call 'political correctness'), Peter Simple, the *Daily Telegraph*'s satirical columnist, created the character of Dr Heinz Kiosk, 'consultant psychiatrist to the Gas Board'. His catch phrase was 'we are all guilty'. A quick read through the chapter titles of this volume would possibly have enraged him still further, but at the same time, suggests to the reader that 'we are all vulnerable' – and that indeed is a useful message to bring before future professionals in the services that support our welfare state. The authors who have contributed to this collective work bring both breadth and depth of knowledge to a tricky subject, and provide sensitive and intelligent thought as well as some striking case studies. Fittingly, since we do not need more blame and despair (which was once the main product of some forms of 'awareness training'), the focus is instead on 'best practice' and some examples are given of models where things have indeed gone right, and lives have been improved. It is good to learn from these as well as being enabled to reflect on our own shortcomings!

We are – as the media have hardly ceased to remind us since the General Election which brought the Coalition Government to power and ended the reign of the 'New' Labour party – living in the era of the 'Big Society'. The theme of this sits well within the traditions of both the post-war Welfare State and also the older traditions of self-reliance coupled with compassion and a religious expectation to care for the weak, enshrined in all known faiths as well as in the mantras of humanism: 'do unto others as you would have them do to (or for) yourself'. In another volume, I have described this as a 'welfare society' (Williams and Johnson 2010). But a welfare society that cares only for those like its perceived majority is by definition not compassionate and inclusive. However, most of us do find it harder to understand or empathize with others who are different – even when those differences are not obviously visible – whether because they derive from sexual orientation, citizenship status, hearing loss or some other 'invisible' impairment, or when they are as distinctive as skin colour, gender or a visible disability. It is not only age that presents us with an involuntary experience of entering 'another country' (Smith 1995).

There is now, very properly, no part of welfare or voluntary work where it is possible to ignore the demands of 'Safeguarding Children' policies and the 'CRB check' is now a routine part of life. However, much less attention seems to have been paid to the needs of people past the transition from childhood to adult life: the 'POVA' (protection of vulnerable adults) regulations are a 'lesser spotted' agenda. However, with developments in the UK Equality Act 2010 and a growing concern for equality and diversity across Europe we all need to be increasingly aware of the risks and rights of all manner of strands of diversity, especially when they overlap or combine. The editors and authors of this book are to be congratulated for producing this text in such a timely fashion, meeting the need to challenge and inform policy and practice through training of new professionals and continuous professional development of the existing workforce. This is more than 'PC' – it has the capacity to improve all our lives.

References

Smith, P. (1995) *Old Age Is Another Country: A Traveler's Guide*. Freedom, CA: Crossing Press.

Williams, C. and Johnson, M.R.D. (2010) *Race and Ethnicity in a Welfare Society*. Maidenhead: Open University Press.

Websites

www.education.gov.uk/childrenandyoungpeople
www.criminalrecordchecks.co.uk
www.equalities.gov.uk
www.fra.europa.eu

PART 1
Explorations in Theory and Practice

Introduction

Margaret Greenfields, Roger Dalrymple and Agnes Fanning

The concept of the 'vulnerable' or 'at-risk' adult has been at the heart of social policymaking in the UK for the past decade. Since the post-war establishment of the welfare state (Lowe 1998), the protection and safeguarding (and more latterly, 're-empowerment' (Johns 2007; Social Care Institute for Excellence 2006) of vulnerable individuals has been a greater or lesser preoccupation of governments of different political complexions. Under the New Labour hegemony of 1997–2010, policymaking in this area gained particular momentum and 'safeguarding' and 'vulnerability' became key words in the political lexicon. Indeed it is greatly to the credit of the former administration that they undertook the first comprehensive review of the plight of vulnerable adults, and introduced a regime which sought to clarify and protect those individuals who are most at risk as a result of their 'status' (e.g. intellectual impairment, mental illness and physical disability, and age-related vulnerability), as hitherto such protection was essentially piecemeal and drawn from a range of differing laws. It is beyond doubt that the concept of mandated protection for adults at risk of harm has in the intervening years become such a core ideal that the idea that in post-modern Britain we should fail to enshrine legislation to adequately protect vulnerable adults appears unthinkably archaic for most students and practitioners in the caring professions.

Despite this consensus of opinion, in the early days of a new coalition administration and in a context of fiscal retrenchment and declining public finance, the discourse around 'at-risk' adults is in the process of being reframed in a broader discussion of the relations between individual and state responsibility for such necessary protective action. Accordingly, social protection initiatives are being re-examined and their efficacy reappraised while practitioners are confronted with dwindling resources with which to fulfil their duties. The time is apt, then, for a book which offers an overview of what it means in practice to work in this important domain in the second decade of the 21st century, and moreover, a text which may be of interest to unpaid carers living with a person at risk or harm, or wider family and friends who are concerned about the well-being of a member of their network who may be a member of a group identified within this volume. Thus, this text includes best practice prescriptions and recommendations which we suggest are valid for carers, family members, students and practitioners working with a variety of at-risk groups in the UK (including those largely invisible groups who may at first glance appear to the busy professional self-sufficient and able to 'care for themselves' such as migrant workers or outwardly confident gay, lesbian, bisexual and transgender co-workers).

So why 'adults at risk of harm', and how do the editors and contributors to this volume conceive of such people and groups? Each political administration nourishes its own policymaking lexicon and the cognate term 'vulnerable', like the often collocated term 'safeguarding', is particularly associated with the Labour administrations of 1997–2010. Indeed the terms are enshrined in a series of central policy documents and legislation of these administrations (e.g. Department of Health and Home Office 2000; Department of Health 2001; Home Office 2006) and have subsequently become key terms across local government, media and academia for discussing and debating the plight of the disadvantaged and socially excluded. While drawing upon the terms 'vulnerable' and 'vulnerability' throughout this book, we generally prefer the description of such adults as 'at risk' as, first, this helps to achieve a certain critical distance from the lexicon of the previous administration and, second, we consider the phrase does greater justice to the dynamic and fluid nature of risk and vulnerability, avoiding the stigma associated with a collective 'label' with overtones of helplessness (Goodley 2000; Smith et al. 2010). The terms 'vulnerability' and 'vulnerable' have been variously defined and interpreted in recent years, with some commentators drawing attention to the contextual nature of vulnerability and others drawing a distinction between actively experienced or *emic* vulnerability, and susceptibility to risk and harm among a particular demographic group – *etic* vulnerability (see further Spiers 2000; Larkin 2009). We consider that the phrase 'at risk' serves well in covering both constituencies and is also helpfully evocative of the exogenous plasticity of disadvantage and exclusion in the post-modern world, synchronizing with the concept of society itself as vulnerable to risk (Beck 1992; Lupton 1999; Wilkinson 2001).

Thus this book provides a rich resource and opportunity for exploration of the challenges and opportunities inherent in working with different constituencies among adults who are at risk of harm. It is designed to be browsed and consulted piecemeal according to the learning needs, personal and professional preoccupations of diverse practitioners in policy, health and social care arenas but it is also amenable to a sequential reading by those who are interested in gaining an overview of the topic of working with adults exposed to particular risks by virtue of status or situation. Indeed, a central theme of the book is the intersectionality of risk and harm: different categories of vulnerability overlap and vulnerable states can open onto each other in a sequent manner (e.g. transition from insecure accommodation to substance abuse and mental ill health to imprisonment). Issues of equality of opportunity and the position of minority communities (who may be excluded on multiple domains as a result of the complex interplay of ethnicity/disability/gender/sexuality) are addressed within the chapters contained herein.

In an attempt to do justice to the dynamic nature of the subject, the materials within this text are organized according to two central principles. The first section presents eight explorations of theory and practice in which an expert practitioner working with a specific vulnerable group provides an overview of the relevant policy context and applies a range of theoretical lenses to the challenges and opportunities for carers, students, academics and practitioners 'in the field'. The organization of this 'Explorations in Theory and Practice' section attempts to reflect the complex and intersectional nature of risk by offering chapters which consider vulnerability at certain stages of the lifespan. Potter (on vulnerable parents, many of whom are themselves young) and Fanning (writing on age-related risk of harm) as well as a further six contributions (Burton, Parris, Mgutshini, Farquharson and Aitken, Greenfields, Cole), explore the ways in which physical and mental impairments, economic advantage, deprivation and social stigma can compound vulnerability at any stage of the life-cycle and allow risk to crystallize into harm. Each of these chapters outline learning objectives for practitioners consulting the book as part of a course of studies, and reflection points for all readers whether they be carers, specialist practitioners or interested generalists who perhaps work in services utilized by numerous diverse groups.

The book's second section gives centre-stage to the narratives of vulnerable adults themselves. Four discrete case-studies (Greenfields, Edwards, Harries and Bailey) capture the experiences, attitudes and perceptions of communities and individuals who are vulnerable as a result of their membership of a class of person. Drawn from the apparently diverse constituencies of Gypsies and Travellers, of individuals who have multiple challenges (impairment, experiences of racism, substance misuse issues and insecure accommodation), the coming-out narratives of lesbian and gay young people and the risks experienced by adult migrants, the case studies again demonstrate the intersectionality of risk and the likelihood that any single 'vulnerable adult' will in fact be at risk of harm in more than one domain over the life-course. We offer this combination of narrative and theory to illustrate the often underestimated complexities and dynamics experienced by those who can all too frequently 'fall through the net' by virtue of their invisibility in discourse around vulnerability, or a gaze which spotlights one particular dimension of their identity and circumstances at the expense of a holistic view (see further Chapter 13, Conclusion).

While the change of UK Government (in May 2010) has lent a distinctly different policy complexion to the formation of numerous state-mandated approaches to societal responsibility, and has already prompted the tentative formation of a new discourse for engaging with concepts of risk and vulnerability within the context of 'the Big Society', it is self-evident that a new set of descriptors will soon have been evolved for engaging with and framing such notions as 'harm', 'risk', 'duty' and 'responsibility' under the auspices of a rapidly changing polity. It is thus helpful to be able to step back from the diversions of political and policymaking discourse to engage with themes of multilayered vulnerabilities in broader, more comprehensive and theorized terms. The text is thus consciously designed to offer both an aid to reflection and to function as a sourcebook for carers and practitioners working in different fields of community practice, health and social care, and to be accessible enough to act as a primer for the general reader seeking a broad overview of social interventions for the vulnerable and socially excluded in the second decade of the 21st century.

Within the conclusion to this book we seek to elaborate a range of perspectives for conceptualizing risk, harm and vulnerability within a fast-moving society, drawing together emergent themes from the preceding chapters and case studies while moving beyond the buzz words and political lexicon of the government of the day. In so doing, it is intended that readers of the conclusion will encounter broader and more theorized notions of how individuals become vulnerable in the matrix of social interaction and of the distribution of resources across diverse social groups, framing an awareness of the 'denial of recognition' (Honneth 1995: 131), which excludes the vulnerable and marginalized individual from recognition as an autonomous, morally responsible and socially valued person. If by perusing this text greater awareness is prompted of the disadvantage facing large swathes of society who are excluded from the (ever-narrowing) purview of 'normative' society then we consider that our work has borne fruit.

References

Beck, U. (1992) *Risk Society: Towards a New Modernity*. London: Sage.

Department of Health (DoH) (2001) *National Plan for Safeguarding Children from Commercial Sexual Exploitation*. London: HMSO.

Department of Health and Home Office (2000) *No Secrets: Guidance on Developing and Implementing Multi-agency Policies and Procedures to Protect Vulnerable Adults from Abuse*, OH Circular HSC 2000/007.

Goodley, D. (2000) *Self-advocacy in the Lives of People with Learning Difficulties: The Politics of Resilience*. Buckingham: Open University Press.

Home Office (2006) *Safeguarding Vulnerable Groups Act 2006*. London: TSO.

Honneth, A. (1995) *The Struggle for Recognition: The Moral Grammar of Social Conflicts*. Cambridge: Polity.

Johns, R. (2007) Who decides now? Protecting and empowering vulnerable adults who lose the capacity to make decisions for themselves. *British Journal of Social Work*, 37(3): 557–64.

Larkin, M. (2009) *Vulnerable Groups in Health and Social Care*. London: Sage.

Lowe, R. (1998) *The Welfare State in Britain Since 1945*. Basingstoke: Macmillan.

Lupton, D. (ed.) (1999) *Risk and Sociocultural Theory: New Directions and Perspectives*. Cambridge: Cambridge University Press.

Smith, M., Bernard, C., Rossiter, K., Sahni, S. and Silva, D. (2010) Vulnerability: a contentious and fluid term. *Hastings Center Report* 40(1): 5–6.

Social Care Institute for Excellence (SCIE) (2006) *Adult Services Practice Guide: Dignity in Care*. London: SCIE.

Spiers, J. (2000) New perspectives on vulnerability using *emic* and *etic* approaches. *Journal of Advanced Nursing*, 31(3): 715–21.

Wilkinson, I. (2001) Social theories of risk perception: at once indispensible and insufficient. *Current Sociology*, 49(1): 1–22.

1 Parenthood

Kate Potter

Over the last decade a significant amount of focus from government and the media has been placed on improving the prospects and outcomes for children. It is clear that to succeed in this there needs to be better support for all families. This chapter focuses on the importance of being aware of the impact of vulnerability on parenting and the professional's role in facilitating access to appropriate help.

Learning objectives

Readers of this chapter will be able to:

- gain a heightened awareness of the skills and knowledge domains involved in working with vulnerable parents;
- recognize the need for an inter-agency approach to supporting parents across both children's and adult services and have an awareness of current policy initiatives being introduced to support better working practices;
- be aware of the impact of poor physical and mental health, disability, and all factors causing exclusion on children and families;
- identify risks to the well-being of children and understand the importance of early interventions to support families to prevent harmful situations arising.

Introduction

Becoming a parent is among the most life-changing events that any person experiences, the actuality of parenthood usually proving much more complex than initially imagined. Media images of idealized early parenthood conflict with the fatigue and stress of the early post-natal period and the challenges which subsequently arise through all stages of childhood and adolescence (Deave et al. 2008). For all new parents, whether they are partnered or alone, the need for support from both the extended family and the wider community should not be underestimated. All mothers need support and guidance as early as possible in pregnancy to ensure that the most positive outcome for the baby in terms of health, well-being and prospects is achieved, research of the last 15 years having shown that from conception, a foetus is affected by both the physical and mental health of the mother (Olds 2006). The need for coherent help and guidance continues as children move from babyhood through young childhood (Gerhardt 2003) and into the teenage years (O'Brien and Scott 2007). It follows that interventions and support strategies for working with vulnerable parents are of central importance in social care provision, the *Reaching Out* document (HM Government 2006) being the most recent of a chain of affirmations of this need. Vulnerability of a parent, whether due to a physical or learning disability, poor mental health or substance abuse, means the family is more likely to be suffering poverty, which often leads to social exclusion and poor access to statutory services (Dearden and Becker 2000).

Accordingly, this chapter considers the areas of awareness and skill sets that practitioners can helpfully develop in supporting and working with vulnerable parents, always remaining mindful of how parental vulnerability impacts on the prospective outcomes for children. For better outcomes for both parent and child, practitioners in health and social care need to gain a coherent and nuanced understanding of the acceptable and purposeful support interventions available to them in working with vulnerable parents. In a contribution to gaining this overview, the chapter will look at professionals' perceptions of vulnerability in parents and will argue for the particular importance for practitioners of promoting awareness among vulnerable parents of attachment and emotional development of the children in their care. These 'best-practice' prescriptions will take full cognisance of the kinds of support requested by vulnerable parents themselves and will consider how this is best provided within an inter-agency context. It is important to consider the role of the professional in providing appropriate support to vulnerable parents but also be in assessing any risk to the child. For as Morris and Wates (2006) have observed, in order for the five outcomes of *Every Child Matters*[1] to be realized, there needs to be recognition across all agencies and by all practitioners that 'these outcomes cannot be achieved without addressing the resources, circumstances and capacity of parents and their wider family and community networks' (2006: xv).

Professionals' perceptions of vulnerability

It could be argued that, in effect, all adults are vulnerable as they become parents, given the myriad new experiences and challenges of the parental role. However, in the context of this chapter, the concept of vulnerability will be narrowed to those definitions arising from the fields of health and social care and the attendant literature. Morris and Wates (2006) give a broad definition of disabled parents as those who have physical and/or sensory impairments, learning difficulties, mental health problems, HIV/AIDS and drug and alcohol problems, though this definition should be expanded to include refugees and asylum seekers, travelling families and those who are homeless because of economic difficulties. Many of these groups will have had some contact with either social care or health services prior to becoming parents and it is likely that during pregnancy or the birth of the child they will receive services from an increasing number of agencies. It is also probable that even at this stage there may be diverging professional perceptions of need and of competence in the parental role (Olsen and Clarke 2003). Judgements on the ability to parent are often made by practitioners from a narrow perspective focusing on the problems which may occur rather than the strengths of the parent. A mother with mild learning difficulties may cause concern to a midwife or health visitor who may focus on her poor literacy ability rather than the fact that she is well focused on the needs of her baby. During pregnancy, for the majority of women, contact with the health services is increased.

Likewise, guidelines and protocols need to be interpreted with care if practitioners are to take full cognisance of the different forms of vulnerability among parents. For example, the National Institute for Health and Clinical Excellence (2008) guidelines recommending a minimum number of medical consultations for pregnant women (ten for a first-time mother with an uncomplicated pregnancy; seven for subsequent births) categorize those in need of additional care as individuals having the following conditions:

- HIV or HBV infection;
- use of recreational drugs;
- psychiatric disorders;
- women who are particularly vulnerable or who lack social support.

Alert health and social care practitioners will reflect that this categorization fails to include women with learning difficulties, sensory impairment, alcohol problems or who may be vulnerable due to residency status. These factors are likely to be less evident to practitioners whose professional remit focuses predominantly on the medical well-being of both mother and child – yet they make up an important part of the wider picture of vulnerable parents. Indeed, careful investigation of parents' circumstances may often reveal that those individuals classified as vulnerable are in fact subject to a number of vulnerabilities. The Social Exclusion Task Force (SETF; 2008) identified families who suffer multiple disadvantages and these include families where:

- no parent in the family is in work;
- no parent has any qualifications;
- the mother has mental health problems;
- at least one parent has a long-standing limiting illness, disability or infirmity; as well as
- those in poor-quality or overcrowded housing.

These can be directly seen to link to disadvantages suffered by any vulnerable adult and it is arguably in this wider family context that vulnerable adults should be viewed by practitioners, the children of these families being at a markedly higher risk of adverse outcomes (Social Exclusion Task Force 2007). It is important for practitioners to consider the impact of a person's vulnerability status on their ability to provide both the necessary social and economic structure for their children beyond the short and medium terms so that timely and appropriate support can be provided.

Supporting vulnerable parents during pregnancy

As is routinely the case in working with vulnerable groups, early interventions are of the highest importance. In the case of supporting vulnerable parents, this translates into supporting expectant parents, and particularly mothers, from the earliest stages of pregnancy onwards. Effects of anxiety, depression and substance abuse and domestic violence need to be recognized and paid as much attention as post-natal depression (Bergner et al. 2008). Adults from vulnerable groups are more likely to practise unhealthy lifestyles including poor diet and smoking. They are also more likely to engage in higher-risk lifestyles, thus increasing the chances of infection with HIV (although this is not transmitted directly to the baby during pregnancy, careful management of the mother is needed especially during labour). Many women become increasingly vulnerable in pregnancy when the risk of domestic violence increases. Within England and Wales all midwives and health visitors routinely discuss domestic violence with mothers and give them the opportunity to disclose any abuse (Department of Health (DoH) 2006). All of these factors heighten the challenges of supporting vulnerable parents.

Moreover, the impact of interventions at this early stage registers not only on the well-being of the expectant parents but on the foetal development and subsequent emotional welfare of the unborn child (Gerhardt 2003; Carter 2008). Substance abuse in pregnancy causes growth and developmental problems for the foetus: infants born to mothers who are taking heroin and other opiates, benzodiazepines and cocaine during their pregnancy are likely to experience severe withdrawal symptoms in the neonatal period and will subsequently require very careful monitoring in the perinatal period, often involving a period of time in a special care baby unit with associated risks for the infant and additional stress for the parents. Likewise, foetal alcohol syndrome can cause facial abnormalities, growth and neurocognitive defects (Mukheyjee et al. 2006) and risks to brain development, the risks being greatest in the first 12 weeks after conception.[2] Poor mental health in a pregnant mother will also adversely impact on the foetus: stress and depression not only increase the risk of low birth weight but studies have shown that increased levels of cortisol in the mother's blood due to stress increases foetal cortisol levels. This results in an infant with higher stress levels during the first years of life (Huizink et al. 2002) who is likely to be fractious and more difficult to care for (Carter 2008).

The need for consistent antenatal care and opportunities to attend preparation classes can therefore be seen as critically important for all vulnerable mothers, yet practitioners must be mindful that services are not always available (Ofsted 2009) and that barriers exist for members of vulnerable groups in accessing these services. A recent study found that late booking for antenatal care was markedly more prevalent in women whose partner was unemployed (Rowe and Garcia 2003) while another establishes that up to 1 per cent of women giving birth in the United Kingdom have accessed no antenatal care at all (Hamlyn et al. 2002), some of these being deaf or visually impaired service users or expectant mothers who do not have English as a first language. Meanwhile mothers with physical disabilities, despite improvement to health centres and hospitals, still find it difficult to attend appointments, and sensory impairment can prevent clear understanding of the consultation process (Disability, Pregnancy and Parenthood 2010). Others who have mental health issues, including those who are abusing alcohol and other substances, may have difficulty registering with a general practitioner and accessing the services to which they are entitled (see Mgutshini in Chapter 4 and Cole in Chapter 7). Frequent changes of address among vulnerable groups mean poor continuity of care and less likelihood of establishing trusting relationships with professionals. Depression, anxiety and severe stress are very isolating and make attending groups with strangers very challenging.

In response to these challenges, midwives in Sure Start Children Centres located in deprived areas have over recent years sought to develop services which are better tailored to the needs of vulnerable parents (Ofsted 2009). Services are increasingly provided within the community in a more relaxed setting than a hospital or GP surgery and there are often other advice services available to help support families. More contact during pregnancy gives the opportunity to identify families where there are problems which are likely to impact both on the developing health of the baby and also on the parenting skills developed in the post-natal period. However, evaluation of some of the projects in the centres still shows that they are failing to reach those who are most vulnerable (Ofsted 2009).

Practitioners thus need to be mindful that the nature of the support required by vulnerable parents in the antenatal period will be very dependent on the cause of their vulnerability. For some, it may be appropriate to facilitate their inclusion in mainstream support and parenting classes and thus provide them with a social support network following the birth. For others they initially may find the social aspect of parenting classes and antenatal clinics quite threatening and may require a more tailored programme of care.

Promoting awareness of attachment among vulnerable parents

For vulnerable parents, the stresses of caring for a small baby in the perinatal period may be confounded by concerns regarding housing, physical illness, relationship problems and social isolation. These very real concerns can distract new parents from considerations of attachment and bonding with their child, yet all new parents need help to understand the importance of their early relationships with their babies. It is imperative to be aware of the significance of the need that infants have for consistent and emotionally responsive care. Bowlby influentially defined attachment as a 'lasting psychological connectedness between human beings' (1969: 194) and stressed that infants need to attach to their primary care giver as a fundamental biological process as they require food and protection for their survival. Babies require someone to provide a secure base from which they can explore the world but will provide them with a safe retreat when the world becomes a threatening place (Prior and Glaser 2006). It follows that infants whose parents are emotionally available for them and help regulate their feelings will develop secure attachments (Gerhardt 2003) and that children who have formed a secure attachment in their early years will have better emotional and behavioural outcomes in childhood and later life (Prior and Glaser 2006).

By contrast, if the caregiver is unable to meet the early emotional needs of the baby, they are likely to develop insecure or disorganized attachments (Ainsworth et al. 1978). Both physical and mental ill-health can mean that a parent is not always emotionally available for their child, especially in the early weeks after birth when stress levels can be particularly high. This then can lead to disordered attachments (Cooper et al. 2005), causing children to struggle with broader socialization initially at school and subsequently in relationships later in life (Prior and Glaser 2006). Parents who have poor mental health, including those who abuse drugs and alcohol, may themselves have attachment disorders. They are particularly likely to need sustained and structured support in developing the caregiver sensitivity and the range of appropriate responses to their child (Prior and Glaser 2006), including management of anxiety – their own as well as their child's. Children of parents who are frightening or frightened are at risk of suffering stress mismanagement in later life (Carter 2008).

In the light of these considerations, it is nevertheless equally important not to assume that vulnerability in an adult will prevent them from forming the appropriate warm relationship with their child. Likewise, the informed practitioner will take account not only of the recommendations of literature and evidence-based guidance, but the views of the service users themselves.

What support do parents want?

The above considerations for practitioners working with vulnerable parents are based largely on practice experience and the published literature but what of the views of vulnerable parents themselves? A study of the views and experiences of disabled parents is informative. In 2000 a Task Force on Supporting Disabled Parents in Their Parenting Role was instigated by the Joseph Rowntree Fund supported by the Department of Health, directors of Social Services, the Disabled Parents Network (DPN) and appropriate voluntary organizations (Morris 2003). The following key findings give a clear understanding of the problems faced by disabled parents when attempting to access services.

- Policies and services concerning adults and/or children are commonly developed without consulting or involving disabled parents.
- Disabled parents find it difficult to access information and advice, advocacy and peer support.
- There are particular problems with the relationship between children's services and adults' community care services. Work is required at both national and local level to create the framework for more appropriate service responses.
- Disabled adults sometimes find it difficult to access their entitlements to support under community care legislation. This can lead to them having to rely on their children for assistance (i.e. their children become 'young carers').
- Although assistance with parenting tasks should be available within the current community care framework, disabled people are often told that they can only access support through children and families services.
- Parents often find they can only get a response from services when things reach a crisis, at which point they can be at risk of losing their children into care.
- Mental health policy and practice does not adequately address the fact that many people with mental health support needs are parents.

- Direct payments can provide the flexible support needed but much work remains to be done to increase the numbers of parents receiving direct payments, particularly those from minority ethnic communities, those with learning difficulties and those with mental health support needs.
- Disabled parents experience unequal access to health (including maternity) and other mainstream services for parents and their children.
- Disability benefits do not take account of the additional costs of parenting for disabled adults.

(Joseph Rowntree Foundation 2003)

One of the most concerning aspects of the above findings is the fact that often legal professionals and those from social care believed that the children would be better off residing with a non-disabled parent, and that they themselves were in need of care rather than assistance (Joseph Rowntree Foundation 2003). This negativity is also sometimes seen within the health service: in obstetric care, some disabled parents reported concerning attitudes to their pregnancy, including pressure to terminate a pregnancy because of health problems and insensitivity of staff who refused to consider the access needs of disabled fathers (Disability, Pregnancy and Parenthood 2010). Many parents felt that the focus of assessments was on their parental 'incapacity' rather on their strengths and ability to provide good care for their children (Morris 2003). Morris (2004) further reported that when vulnerable adults wish to be involved in their children's education they face two main barriers: unhelpful or negative attitudes, and access and communication difficulties. Schools will frequently send information by letter which does not acknowledge that parents may have poor or non-existent literacy skills or who do not understand written English. They can then often be labelled as non-caring and unmotivated as parents.

A study carried out on parents living in poor environments by the Policy Research Bureau (Ghate and Hazel 2004) uncovered similar trends, finding that there was often a deficit of services and information available to parents within their own local areas. These parents were also concerned about asking for social support on account of fear of interference and loss of privacy as well as having their lives controlled. Although the parents in this study were not designated as vulnerable or disabled, those who have disabilities are more likely to be affected by economic disadvantage (Cabinet Office 2006). A study by Olsen and Clarke (2003) looked at disabled parents and their families and the role of formal and informal networks in their lives. The parents discussed the importance of doing the ordinary things that all parents want to do with their children, such as taking them out and engaging with their education. They also felt the need for practical and emotional support for parenting and the opportunity for a break from the children occasionally. In the families identified by this study, there were often greater barriers to obtaining the support required. The main issues identified were inaccessibility or failure of adaptation to housing, lack of transport and negative attitudes to themselves as parents (Quinton 2004). Parents, especially those with learning difficulties, reported feeling undermined by practitioners who adopted an attitude of 'the professional knows best' (Booth 2003: 205).

The findings of these studies provide a salutary reminder to practitioners of the need to take account of service users' own views and experiences. There is clearly a greater need to be more responsive to the individual requirements of vulnerable parents, providing support in a timely fashion, respecting parents' strengths and working better across agencies, in the health, social care and the voluntary sector.

Vulnerability in the wider family unit: children and young people as carers

Holistic support for vulnerable parents should also take account of the wider family circumstances and should recognize that in many families where there is a vulnerable parent, children and young people may themselves be required to take on a burden of care and responsibility which is difficult for both parent and child. This pattern was recognized in a 2007 government vision of transforming adult services which encouraged practitioners to work in each instance towards sustaining 'a family unit which avoids children being required to take on inappropriate caring roles' (HM Government 2007: 3). Indeed, of the six million carers in the UK at present (Carers UK 2011) a significant number will be children who care for parents and siblings with both physical and mental health problems. The majority of those needing care are lone parents and these are usually mothers. The help provided by these young carers includes domestic help in the home but 48 per cent also provide general and nursing-type care. Eighty-two per cent provide support of an emotional nature and supervise those they are caring for in some capacity. Intimate care is provided by 18 per cent and 11 per cent also provide child care. Girls are more involved with the tasks of caring and their input increases as they get older. The time spent caring was significant, with 16 per cent spending over 20 hours a week caring. There has been an improvement on the impact of caring on education but 27 per cent are still experiencing problems. Children and young people who care for parents who misuse drugs and alcohol are reported to have more educational difficulties (Dearden and Becker 2004). Parental substance abuse requires young carers to be particularly resilient. The children manage best if they have a good relationship with friends and the wider family but the substance abuse will often mean that the relationship with their parent becomes very difficult. They will frequently also attempt to protect and influence their parent's actions in the hope of stopping the harmful behaviour (Joseph Rowntree Foundation 2004).

It is important to recognize that each young carer will experience different problems dependent on the disability of their parent. Parents with mental health issues, including substance abuse, may struggle to give consistent emotional support and the child will need to establish support networks elsewhere. The impact of having a caring role means that they have less opportunity to mix with their peers and move into adult responsibilities too soon. Reports have shown that a strong personal relationship with a service worker can be of great value (Joseph Rowntree Foundation 2003; Dearden and Becker 2004) but, even more importantly, a strong connection with a family member is most protective (Newman 2003). The need for services to be provided in a timely fashion to prevent family and relationship breakdown is vital to ensure that young carers are able to develop emotionally and achieve in education. It is also important to consider that many children are able to cope in the caring role and proceed successfully into adulthood (Joseph Rowntree Foundation 2004). This emphasizes the need for practitioners to be aware of pressures on all the family.

The *Young Carers Report* (Dearden and Becker 2004) shows that there have already been improvements, with more carers being assessed for need and the growth in the number of Young Carers projects. The current projects are now in contact with 25,000 young carers (HM Government 2008). Recent legislation from the government (HM Government 2007) is aiming to improve the situation and as provision for adult care expands extra help should reach these young people. These provisions, hopefully, will all help to improve the situation for families where more support is needed. Many young carers are concerned that any help will come only via assessment processes and this may result in them or their siblings being taken into care (Barrett 2008). Children and families need to feel secure in order to ask for help and that the family will not be judged adversely or separated. Adequate support and respite where appropriate are likely to improve the family relationships with better outcomes for all the family.

Support for parents: an inter-agency approach

The last decade has seen an increasing emphasis on providing support for parents in the health and social care sectors. The recognition that all parents require support to provide the appropriate environment to ensure that children develop to their full potential is acknowledged in all of the last administration's key policy documents focusing on children administration (Department for Education and Skills (DfES)/DoH 2006; Department for

Children, Schools and Families (DCSF) 2007; DfES 2007; SETF 2007; DoH 2009). Many vulnerable adults may be in contact with various statutory and non-statutory services for their own health or social needs. When they become parents they will be in contact with health practitioners delivering the Child Health Promotion Programme (DoH 2009). This initially will be the General Practitioner and the midwife and following the birth the Health Visiting team. These services will be in addition to any service provision that they already receive. At the age of three, most children will be able to access nursery education through Early Years provision, and the family will be in contact with yet another agency. Research has shown that systems and services for families where there may be added problems are highly complex and fragmented (SETF 2007). The concerns are that accountability may fall between services, that there is a lack of co-ordination between services and often one professional only has a particular view of the family. There are also worries about different thresholds across agencies and this can often hinder good working together (DCSF 2009a, 2009b). Efforts to improve the parental experience and achieve better outcomes for the whole family are being addressed by recent policy. Within the majority of these policies there is an acknowledgement that effective implementation requires partnership working across agencies. The then Department for Children, Schools and Families (DCSF) legislated for the setting-up of Children's Trusts within each local area. The purpose of these Trusts is to ensure cooperation and partnership arrangements between all local agencies to improve the outcomes for children and young people (DCSF 2007). Part of the provision in each area will be Sure Start Children's Centres and extended schools. Although the aim is to reach all children, the emphasis is for a particular focus on the disadvantaged. Sure Start Centres in the 30 per cent most disadvantaged areas will provide extensive child care and early learning facilities for 48 weeks of the year, parenting support and parental outreach and Child and Family health services.[3] The Early Intervention team in their published report continue to support the importance of providing targeted support for the most vulnerable families through the early years (Allen 2011).

Extended school provision will also include childcare provision and parenting support and there is an expectation of easy access to specialist services for families from early years through to secondary schools. These Centres are excellent examples of cross-agency working. Health, education and social care work together and have therefore the opportunity to build strong alliances and a better understanding of the skills and services available across agencies. Similar provision can be found in Scotland through the Early Years Framework.

This vision is admirable and will certainly be valuable for many families. There is concern, however, that the most disadvantaged families may still be excluded from these services. Assessments of the impact on children and their families have shown that although there is integrated working and stronger links are being developed with the voluntary sectors, there is clear evidence that they are still not gaining confidence with the most vulnerable families in the community (Ofsted 2009). Although children's services are taking great strides in working together, it is important to acknowledge that vulnerable parents may be receiving services from agencies that have no focus on children. These families may also be the least likely to engage with services provided in the Children Centres (Ofsted 2009). The *Hidden Harm Report* (Advisory Council on the Misuse of Drugs 2003) established that 350,000 children in the United Kingdom have drug-addicted parents and one million live in a family where one parent is addicted to alcohol. At present treatment services for adults are under no legal requirement to establish whether there are any dependent children (Carter 2008). It is therefore possible that families which need support because of substance abuse may not receive support from children's services until crisis point has been reached. Adult disability and mental health services need to have a more holistic approach to providing care for their clients, and be aware of the impact of the illness and disability on all the family (Barrett 2008). Examples of good practice can be found across the country emanating from the government-funded Family Pathfinders programme (DCSF 2007). A whole family package of support is provided by a team consisting of practitioners from both adult and children services working together (DCSF 2010b).

The importance of sharing information across agencies to protect both vulnerable adults and their children has been underlined in reports and policy documents throughout the decade (DCSF 2009a; HM Government 2010). In line with professional codes of conduct, practitioners are rightly concerned to protect the confidentiality of the clients or service users they are engaged with. There is also the need to maintain the trust of the client or service user and a concern that this may be jeopardized by involving another discipline or agency. Best practice is to be open and honest with the client and give clear reasons as to why the information needs to be shared and with whom. Practitioners need to be provided with support and guidance from their managers to ensure that the information shared is necessary, proportionate, relevant, accurate, timely and secure (DCSF 2008). It is important that all decisions regarding information sharing are recorded so that the rationale for that decision is clearly demonstrated. The provisions of the Children Act (2004) also required all Local Authorities to provide access to the Contact Point Database to authorized practitioners working in education, health and social care (DCSF 2010a, 2010b). Implementation was started but found to be very expensive. There were also concerns that human rights might be breached so the project has now been abandoned. However, this does not absolve all practitioners from the responsibility of ensuring that information relevant to the well-being of families is shared effectively across agencies.

Scenario for reflection

Fran (aged 35) and Greg (aged 42) have been married for 16 years. They have three children Becky (aged 14), Simon (aged 12) and Clare (aged 2). They live in a three-bedroom council property. Fran suffered severe post-natal depression after the birth of Clare and has been diagnosed with ME (myalgic encephalopathy) in the last six months. She is unable to walk unaided and can do very little around the house or care for the children. Greg lost his job as a driver for a local haulage company at about the same time. He has been caring for the family but has started to drink very heavily and is no longer engaging with the children.

Consider:

- what are the implications for each member of the family?
- how can services, both statutory and voluntary, work together to improve outcomes for the family?

Working together to identify risk

Throughout this chapter it has been evident that vulnerable parents may need to receive additional support at any stage from early pregnancy through to late adolescence. This may be required for myriad reasons including a worsening of a parent's disability or a deterioration in their mental health, a family breakdown, bereavement or loss of home or employment. A focus for any risk will be on the children rather than the parent. The need of the child, is by necessity, paramount (DCSF 2009b). The process of assessment can enable parents to identify specific issues which are impacting on their children and how support can best be provided to keep the family together. The *Common Assessment Framework* (CAF) remains one of the central elements of government strategy for better integration of children's services (DfES 2004). The vision of the previous administration was that practices and services would be determined by the needs of children and families rather than the constraints of professional boundaries. The concept is that one assessment can be carried out and shared by a lead professional across all agencies, thus avoiding the multiple and overlapping assessments often experienced by families with complex needs. Early evaluation (Brandon et al. 2006) shows that the process works best when initial assessment is carried out by the concerned practitioner rather than passed on to another professional or agency. For vulnerable families, where there already may be a practitioner from health or social care supporting the parent, it is sensible that they complete the CAF referral with the family. This practitioner is likely to have the most in-depth under-standing of the family's situation and possibly the most trusting relationship.

Adult workers may not have a great understanding of child health and development but will often be very aware of the family and environmental issues, and working alongside the parent, will be aware of persistent or new and emerging problems which may impact on their parenting ability. The aim of the CAF is to identify children who require support in addition to those provided by the universal services. A key worker known to the family will be in the ideal situation to explain the CAF process and help the family identify what support they need in order to achieve the best outcomes for their children. The research identifies that referrals are often left until a severe crisis occurs (Social Care Institute for Excellence (SCIE) 2005).

All practitioners need to recognize when children are not just in need but may be at risk of significant harm (DfES 2006). This recognition may be diffi-cult for practitioners who have developed good working relationships with vulnerable adults and they may find challenging them about their parenting capacity very difficult. Following the death of Baby Peter in 2007, Lord Laming produced a report focusing on the progress being made in safeguarding the health and well-being of children (Laming 2009). He identified both good practice and barriers across all agencies in providing services to adequately protect children. One recommendation was that all police, probation, adult mental health and adult drug and alcohol services have a well-understood referral process when there are serious concerns regarding the safety of a child. The high profile obtained by a number of serious case reviews over the last year has increased awareness among all professionals working with families. The impact on children's services has been considerable. Although initial referrals have only increased by 2 per cent the number of children who are the subject of a child protection plan is up by 17 per cent, and those entering the care system by 9 per cent (HM Government 2010). The hope is that these child protection plans are appropriate and meet the needs of the families involved. Raised awareness is needed by all practitioners (Laming 2009) but practitioners should always act in the best interest of the child and consider whether their actions constitute defensive practice. There is statistical evidence that children of parents with learning difficulties and those who have mental health prob-lems are at a high risk of entering the care system (Booth 2003; SCIE 2009). Goodinge (2000) discusses evidence that parents with learning disabilities are particularly disadvantaged and are often assessed with an over-zealous attitude to risk. It can be argued that this attitude leads to injustice in family courts and the care system towards parents with learning disabilities (Booth 2003). Practitioners from children's services need to have a greater understanding of learning disability and mental health in order to make an informed decision as to risks to children (SCIE 2009). This calls for more joint training across all services (SCIE 2009) and a greater discussion around parenting capability with all practitioners. It is then hoped that more support can be provided earlier to prevent crisis (Laming 2009). All practitioners working with vulnerable parents need to help them engage with services which are appropriate for their family. They can advocate for the parents and help other agencies understand what works best for them. A practitioner in adult mental health is often better placed to judge best how to engage parents with children's services. They also need to be supported in their work with parents who are failing to engage with these services and be aware of the risk that this refusal may pose to the children (HM Government 2010). Figure 1.1 shows a plan of assessment of parenting capacity and family risk.

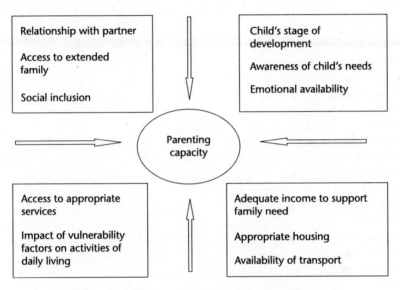

Figure 1.1   Assessment of parenting capacity and family risk.

Conclusion

The provision of emotional and physical support and protection for their children is a challenge for all parents, these challenges being greatly exacerbated for those from vulnerable groups. While all parents require support to make the best provision for their children, vulnerable adults when they become parents often face greater barriers in accessing appropriate support. These barriers may be physical or attitudinal but the outcome of not receiving appropriate support will be to place additional strain upon the vulnerable parent and to adversely affect the child. As suggested by the preceding discussion, there has been a growing recognition in research and government policy that early intervention is vital to prevent escalation of the problems faced by vulnerable parents. All practitioners working with such parents need to assess the wider family in a holistic and non-judgemental manner. They need to understand the impact of the parent's disability or mental ill-health on their ability to parent and to assist parents in accessing the support they need in a timely fashion to prevent a subsequent need for crisis intervention. Better communication, both with families and across services, should be developed. Services need to support their staff with clear guidelines on appropriate information sharing which will benefit their service users. Services provided should be adapted to the specific need of the family and should recognize and value the strengths of the parents as well as identifying areas where support is needed. This model of partnership working is best placed to address the needs of vulnerable parents and to support the induction of their children into a life where their own prospects for escaping life's vulnerabilities are maximized.

Chapter summary

- All parents require support to achieve the best outcomes for their children.
- Different stages of development in children will place different pressures on parents and this needs to be considered when assessing what support is required.
- Vulnerable adults frequently face greater barriers in accessing support through disability or social exclusion.
- Practitioners' perceptions of ability to parent can often be highly judgemental and not focused on the best outcomes for the whole family. Focus should be on strengths rather than weaknesses.
- Although great strides have been taken in integrated working across services to help families, there is still clear evidence that there are deficits in communication.

Notes

1   *Every Child Matters: Change for Children* (DfES 2004) provided the framework to maximize opportunity and minimize risk for all children focusing on the five key outcomes of being healthy, staying safe, enjoying and achieving, making a positive contribution and achieving economic well-being. The present government has replaced the five outcomes with the goal to 'help children achieve more' (HM Government 2010).

2   In unplanned pregnancies many women will be unaware that they are
    pregnant until eight to twelve weeks and may continue with behaviours
    putting the foetus at risk (British Medical Association Board of Science 2007).
3   Since the Coalition Government took office in May 2010 the Department
    of Education now has responsibility for Children's Services. At the time
    of writing there have been no major changes in policies affecting these
    services. There are concerns, however, that cuts within local authority budgets
    will impinge on service provision.

References

Advisory Council on the Misuse of Drugs (2003) *Hidden Harm: Responding to the Needs of Children of Problem Drug Users*. London: Advsisory Council on the Misuse of Drugs.

Ainsworth, M., Blehar, M., Waters, E. and Wall, S. (1978) *Patterns of Attachment: A Psychological Study of the Strange Situation*. Mahwah, NJ: Erlbaum.

Allen, G. (2011) *Early Interventions: The Next Steps*. London: HM Government.

Barrett, H. (2008) *'Hard to Reach' Families: Engagement in the Voluntary and Community Sector*. London: Family and Parenting Institute.

Bergner, S., Monk, C. and Werner, E. (2008) Dyadic intervention during pregnancy? Treating pregnant women and possibly reaching the future baby. *Infant Mental Health Journal*, 29(5): 399–419.

Booth, T. (2003) Parents with learning difficulties and the stolen generation. *Journal of Learning Disability*, 7(3): 203–9.

Bowlby, J. (1969) *Attachment and Loss: Volume 1 Attachment*. London: Hogarth Press.

Brandon, M., Howe, A., Dagley, V., Salter, C., Warren, C. and Black, J. (2006) *Evaluating the Common Assessment Framework and Lead Professional Guidance and Implementation in 2006: Research Report*. London: DfES.

British Medical Association Board of Science (2007) *Fetal Alcohol Spectrum Disorder: A Guide for Health Professionals*. London: BMA.

Cabinet Office (2006) *Reaching Out: An Action Plan on Social Exclusion*. London: The Cabinet Office.

Carers UK (2011) *Valuing Carers: Calculating the Value of Carers' Support*. London: Carers UK.

Carter, S. (2008) *The Next Generation: A Policy Report from the Early Years Commission*. London: Centre for Social Justice.

Cooper, M., Hooper, C. and Thompson, M. (eds) (2005) *Child and Adolescent Mental Health Theory and Practice*. London: Hodder Arnold.

Dearden, C. and Becker, S. (2000) *Growing up Caring: Vulnerability and Transition to Adulthood – Young Carers' Experiences*. Leicester: Youth Work Press/Joseph Rowntree Foundation.

Dearden, C. and Becker, S. (2004) *Young Carers in the UK*. London: Carers UK.

Deave, T., Johnson, D. and Ingram, J. (2008) *Transition to Parenthood: The Needs of Parents in Pregnancy and Early Parenthood*. Bristol: Centre for Child and Adolescent Health, University of West of England.

Department for Children, Schools and Families (DCSF) (2007) *The Children's Plan: Building Brighter Futures*. London: DCSF.

Department for Children, Schools and Families (DCSF) (2008) *Information Sharing: Guidance for Practitioners and Managers*. London: DCSF.

Department for Children, Schools and Families (DCSF) (2009a) *Working Together to Safeguard Children*. London: DCSF.

Department for Children, Schools and Families (DCSF) (2009b) *Common Assessment Framework: Practitioners Guide*. London: DCSF.

Department for Children, Schools and Families (DCSF) (2010a) *Contact Point Fact Sheet*. London: DCSF.

Department for Children, Schools and Families (DCSF) (2010b) *Think Family Pathfinders: Research Update*. London: DCSF.

Department for Education and Skills (DfES) (2004) *Every Child Matters: Change for Children*. London: DfES.

Department for Education and Skills (DfES) (2006) *What to Do if You Are Worried a Child Is Being Abused*. London: DfES.

Department for Education and Skills (DfES) (2007) *Governance Guidance for Sure Start Children's Centres and Extended Schools*. London: DfES.

Department for Education and Skills/Department of Health (2006) *Joint Planning and Commissioning Framework for Children, Young People and Maternity Services* London: DfES/DoH.

Department of Health (DoH) (2000) *Framework for the Assessment of Children in Need and Their Families*. London: Department of Health.

Department of Health (DoH) (2004) *National Service Framework for Children, Young People and Maternity Services*. London: Department of Health.

Department of Health (DoH) (2006) *Domestic Violence: A Resource Manual for Healthcare Professionals*. London: Department of Health.

Department of Health (DoH) (2009) *The Child Health Promotion Programme*. London: Department of Health.

Disability, Pregnancy and Parenthood (2010) *The Maternity Information Gap for Physically Disabled People*. http://www.dppi.org.uk/projects/episurvey.php.

Gerhardt, S. (2003) *Why Love Matters*. London: Routledge.

Ghate, D. and Hazel, N. (2004) *Parenting in Poor Environments: Stress, Support and Coping*. London: Policy Research Bureau.

Goodinge, S. (2000) *A Jigsaw of Services: Inspection of Services to Support Disabled Adults in Their Parenting Role*. London: SCIE DoH.

Hamlyn, B., Brooker, S., Oleinikova K. and Wanda, S. (2002) *Infant Feeding 2000*. London. HMSO.

Her Majesty's Government (2006) *Reaching Out: An Action Plan for Social Exclusion*. London: Cabinet Office.

Her Majesty's Government (2007) *Putting People First: A Shared Vision and Commitment to the Transformation of Adult Care.* London: Department of Health.

Her Majesty's Government (2008) *Carers at the Heart of 21st-century Families and Communities.* London: Department of Health.

Her Majesty's Government (2010) *The Government's Response to Lord Laming: One Year On.* London: HM Government.

Huizink, A., Robles De Medina, P., Mulder, E., Visser, G. and Buiteler, J. (2002) Psychological measures of prenatal stress as predictors of infant temperament. *Journal of the American Academy of Child and Adolescent Psychiatry*, 41(9): 1078–81.

Joseph Rowntree Foundation (2003) *Findings: Supporting Disabled Adults in Their Parenting Role.* York: Joseph Rowntree Foundation.

Joseph Rowntree Foundation (2004) *Findings: The Effect of Parental Substance Abuse on Young People.* York: Joseph Rowntree Foundation.

Laming, W. (2009) *The Protection of Children in England: A Progress Report.* London: DFCS.

Morris, J. (2003) *The Right Support: Report of the Task Force on Supporting Disabled Adults in Their Parenting Role.* York: Joseph Rowntree Foundation.

Morris, J. (2004) *Disabled Parents and Schools: Barriers to Parental Involvement in Children's Education.* York: Joseph Rowntree Foundation.

Morris, J. and Wates, M. (2006) *Supporting Disabled Parents and Parents with Additional Support Needs.* London: SCIE.

Mukheyjee, R., Hollins, S. and Turk, J. (2006) Fetal alcohol spectrum disorder: an overview. *The Royal Society of Medicine*, 99: 298–302.

National Institute for Health and Clinical Excellence (NICE) (2008) *Antenatal Care: Routine Care for the Healthy Pregnant Woman.* London: NICE.

Newman, T. (2003) *Children of Disabled Parents.* Lyme Regis: Russell House.

O'Brien, C. and Scott, J. (2007) The role of the family in J Coleman and A Hagell (eds) *Adolescence, Risk and Resilience: Against the Odds.* Chichester: Wiley.

Ofsted (2009) *The Impact of Integrated Services on Children and Their Families in Sure Start Children's Centres.* London: Ofsted.

Olds, D. (2006) The nurse–family partnership: an evidence-based preventative intervention. *Infant Mental Health Journal*, 27(1): 5–25.

Olsen, R. and Clarke, H. (2003) *Parenting and Disability: Disabled Parents' Experiences of Raising Children.* Bristol: Policy Press.

Prior, V. and Glaser, D. (2006) *Understanding Attachment and Attachment Disorder.* London: Jessica Kingsley.

Quinton, D. (2004) *Supporting Parents: Messages from Research.* London: Jessica Kingsley.

Rowe, R. and Garcia, J. (2003) Social class, ethnicity and attendance for antenatal care in the United Kingdom: a systematic review. *Journal of Public Health Medicine*, 25(2): 113–19.

Social Care Institute for Excellence (SCIE) (2005) *Helping Parents with Learning Disabilities in Their Role as Parents.* London: SCIE.

Social Care Institute for Excellence (SCIE) (2009) *Think Child, Think Parent, Think Family: A Guide to Parental Mental Health and Child Welfare.* London: SCIE.

Social Exclusion Task Force (SETF) (2007) *Reaching Out: Think Family.* London: The Cabinet Office.

Social Exclusion Task Force (SETF) (2008) *Families at Risk.* London: The Cabinet Office.

Sunderland, M. (2006) *The Science of Parenting.* London: Dorling Kindersley.

2 Physical disability

Jennifer Burton

This chapter explores physical and associated disabilities within the context of policy approaches and legislation which have directly influenced the ways that disabled adults live their lives today. Emphasis will be placed on an exploration of the impact of life opportunities for disabled people within a society experiencing financial, social and emotional pressures as well as the direct effect of multi-factorial disabilities and intersectional risk which can escalate into oppression, exclusion, risk of exploitation and abuse. The association between cultural issues and experiences of disability from a historical and contemporary perspective will be explored and the factors which may have a significant influence on disabled people within society, causing them to be vulnerable to risk of abuse, will be identified. Abuse will be referred to in its broadest sense, rather than a narrow legal definition and will be considered as a continuum based upon the individual circumstances, degree of vulnerability of the person, risks of harm and their frequency as well as the person's capacity to consent.

Learning objectives

Readers of this chapter will be able to:

- consider different life experiences for disabled people in contemporary society and how harm can escalate into risk and abusive situations;
- set the current experiences of disabled people within the context of a historical, social and political framework;
- explore power differentials between disabled and non-disabled people from different perspectives, including those of service users, carers, feminist and disability movements;
- consider definitions of abuse and the personal experiences of people whose lives have been directly affected by the impact of abuse and exploitation.

In exploring physical disability and vulnerability, this chapter will progress from an initial, brief historical overview, marking the deep-rooted cultural impact of disability discrimination and abuse which has evolved over generations and still implicit in modern-day life. This will refer to the situation across Britain in the 19th century, although later references to policy and legislation around safeguarding adults will exclude Scotland, as the legislative framework has differed to that in the rest of Britain. The historical context will then be reinforced by a brief overview of the socio-political factors which have shaped adult social care today.

The changing features of abuse and dominating factors influenced by changes in the way we live will also be explored. A feature of abuse which is increasing is discriminatory abuse experienced by people who may be vulnerable due to their disability who now live in their own homes and may be an easy target for exploitation. The reasons why people abuse will also be explored, to consider the triggers for abusive relationships and how these can be prevented. Emphasis will be placed on the experiences of people with multiple disabilities in an attempt to unpack the complex layering of influences impacting on a person's well-being. For example, a person with an enduring health problem such as diabetes and a physical disability, who is also an asylum seeker in the UK is likely to experience a range of difficulties and possible discrimination due to the multiple impact of struggling through the maze of benefit entitlement, language barriers and personal and cultural differences.

Finally, the chapter will identify some of the positive responses to safeguarding vulnerable adults from abuse which encompasses new and protective legislation, the disability movement and a developing ideology across social care professions to recognize and aim to combat abuse by working towards shared values and non-oppressive practices.

An historical perspective

There is a rich and powerful history in Britain which provides a picture of how individuals with a disability have been displaced and estranged from mainstream society over a very long period of time. Although local history can differ, the details of the impact of early legislation and how it was administered are essentially the same in all parts of the United Kingdom. The Poor Law Amendment Act in 1834 which extended its power from the original Poor Law of the 16th century established the criteria for eligibility to people made destitute due to their disabilities (largely understood in these contexts as physical impairment). A network of workhouses was created all over the country which shifted the responsibility for care away from public relief funds for families to moving disabled people away from their families and local communities into the workhouses. The mid-19th century saw a massive development of charity or mission work which resulted in many vulnerable people being housed in religious institutions, asylums, hospitals or workhouses. By 1840 there were a staggering 28,880 charities and the emergence of famous middle-class philanthropists and reformers, such as Elizabeth Fry, Florence Nightingale and Dr Barnardo, who shaped the emerging welfare systems. By 1930 the administration of the Poor Law was taken over by elected local authorities, who appropriated more than half of the workhouses as hospitals. The shift from voluntary and charitable works towards the medical model of service delivery increased as the medical profession became responsible for the admission to the hospital wards. The National Health Service Act in 1946 and the newly emerging Health Service inherited around 55,000 hospital beds which were designated for the chronically sick (Pater 1981).

The decision-making process distinguishing between those with the power and ability to be accepted into ordinary life and those who were disempowered due to their disability and displaced to live apart from mainstream society is a central thread running through this journey through time. The enduring impact of the time line of history on contemporary life experiences for disabled people cannot be denied, yet it is difficult to fully understand the continuing influences. Foucault wrote about the power differences which have shaped history to maintain inequalities across different groups (Danaher 2000). The divide between the powerful and the oppressed is referred to by Foucault as the 'order of things'; the ideology reinforcing power as a complex flow of relations between groups and sections of society. The ideas created by people become truths which are not natural but are produced in order to 'support, advantage or valorise a particular social group' (Danaher 2000: 9).

The ideology of disability and implicit references to oppression and denial can be seen to be directly linked to prejudice stemming from the stereotypes created by society which then ranks people into a 'hierarchy of being'. This concept can be linked with the concept of 'patriarchy' which translated means 'the law of the father' (Weber 1947). Its use has been extended to refer to the dominance of men and the uneven distribution of power in society. The idea of male power also link with capitalism and the Marxist ideas of men as 'producers' and women as 'nurturers' (Rowbotham 1973). The notion of a hierarchy within humankind can be seen to go a step further and perceive that people with a physical disability may hold less power because they may be outside the 'norm' of independent and fully functioning adults able to contribute financially and socially within society. The ideas of difference have been linked with innate values about what is 'normal' and what is 'abnormal'. In the 19th century, visual differences became very important for measuring and categorizing physical and intellectual anomalies. This was heightened by the invention of photography. Cesare Lombroso (1911) became well known for categorizing physical characteristics which were supposed to signify mental disability, mental illness, immorality and criminality; 'one slipping easily into the other' (Sibley 1995: 25). A series of black and white photographs in this text show Cesare Lombroso's use of photographic portraits in his work on criminality and madness, demonstrating the importance of physical categorization in the cultural construction of normality and deviance (Ferrero 1911).

These images of difference could be seen to lend themselves to theories of disablism and racism which were magnified in Nazi Germany where Jews, defined in terms of physical difference or 'imperfection', became 'dangerous', as did people with learning and physical disabilities due to the ideological belief of a threat to the purity and the stability of the Aryan race.[1] A piece of history that is seldom recognized is that gas chambers were first invented to kill large numbers of people with learning difficulties, before the development of the technology for the mass killing of Jews. The 'euthanasia' of disabled people on a large scale was an extension of the programme introduced by the Nazis in 1933, only six months after they came to power in Germany, to sterilize the 'hereditarily' sick. This programme is thought to have resulted in the forced sterilization of 21,000 people with physical impairments, 20,000 with sensory impairments, 60,000 with epilepsy, 100,000 people with mental health problems and 200,000 people with learning difficulties (Williams 2006).

Reflection on practice

Considering contemporary experiences for disabled people, what barriers may still be in place in society which may require a disabled person to seek support and advice from different services and professionals?

You may have thought of several barriers, such as difficulties in accessing public buildings, public transport, the need for aids and adaptations to be able to gain entry to employment, leisure and social opportunities that may otherwise be denied them. Other barriers experienced may include risk of isolation and exclusion causing mental health problems and financial dependency on welfare benefits if employment expectations are not achievable.

This brief exploration of history has gathered together some of the powerful experiences of disabled people through a time line of evolving ideas and changing values which have direct links with key socio-political directives.

Policy and impact on practice

The Disability Discrimination Act (1995) defines disability as encompassing a wide spectrum of conditions, ranging from physical, learning and sensory disabilities through to people with chronic illness, medical conditions and mental health issues. Therefore, 'disability' is an umbrella term which increases the number of conditions considered to be disabling all the time, and can be summed up as a negative experience in one or more dimensions of impairment, which limit or restrict participation in life experiences. The interplay of multiple disabilities, life chances and adversity, the benefit or absence of family bonds and support networks can all be contributing factors as to whether a person becomes vulnerable to risk and harm, or is able to retain their individuality due to personal resilience and ability to cope with the pressures of life.

There is a tenuous link between disability and vulnerability which is arguably emphasized by current government-driven legislation. An accepted definition of what constitutes a vulnerable adult stems from Department of Health policies (in 2000) which adopted the Law Commission definition as follows:

> anyone of 18 years and over who is or may be in need of community care services by reason of mental or other disability, age or illness and who is or may be unable to take care of himself or herself, or unable to protect himself or herself against significant harm or serious exploitation.
>
> (Brown 2010: 114)

An important focus is the factors that can result in a person with a physical disability becoming vulnerable. These factors have altered considerably as society has moved from excluding groups of people with disabilities from mainstream society towards a more inclusive philosophy influenced by socio-political ideas, based on the value of individuality and difference. The risk factors have altered rather than disappeared, however, and will be considered as part of the next section addressing types of risk linked to harm and abuse.

Although the vast majority of physically disabled people are able to live ordinary lives and through personal resilience and family support are able to cope with their disabilities, there are others who are considered to be eligible for social care support. *Fair Access to Care Services* guidance (DoH 2002) requires that an assessment of needs is carried out and the eligible needs are then prioritized. These eligible needs are defined in terms of risk and categorized in terms of 'critical', 'substantial', 'moderate' or 'low' bands of need. Cambridge and Carnaby (2005) have argued that this approach is narrow and removes the potential for preventative work which may reduce risks of vulnerability and increase independence and quality of life for disabled people requiring lower levels of support, which are unlikely to be met due to the priority being placed on those with critical or substantial levels of need. The reasons for disabled individuals requiring support are many and varied, ranging from advancing age, poverty, the loss of a main carer, unemployment, mental illness, alcohol or drug abuse.

Legislative responses to managing the way that local authorities support people who are vulnerable due to their disability has shifted from a block contract approach using traditional day, residential and nursing services towards the personalization of support. The *Putting People First: A Shared Vision and Commitment to the Transformation of Adult Social Care* (DoH 2007) promoted self-directed support and personal budgets for those eligible for publicly funded adult social care, with family carers having a significant role as care partners.

Early consultation linked with a pilot to monitor the first individual budgets (National Evaluation of the Individual Budgets Pilot Programme, October 2008) has flagged up concerns about increases in abuse linked to personal care being provided in people's own homes. Early indications identified that younger physically disabled people who had experienced an individual budget found this very empowering and managed the transition to receiving support in their own home well. There is concern, however, that, with the ethos of individuals having their support within their own or their family home, that abuse may increase. The focus will be on self-assessment rather than the traditional community care assessment, and individuals will use the allocated individual budget to employ their own personal carer. This may be a family member, friend or relative. The challenge in supporting this model of care may be the need to recognize the increased benefits, control and autonomy that is afforded to the individual and also the increased risks of ordinary living. There is a fine line between personal care and poor care, and between personal autonomy and neglect.

Risk factors linked or leading to harm and abuse

One of the recurring messages in contemporary adult support services has been the impact of the financial recession across the UK. There have been implicit references to a linked social and psychological recession, triggered by the wide-scale impact of the credit crunch. There appear to be a wide range of issues emerging as a result of an increasing number of people disadvantaged by life in the UK today and experiencing financial, social and emotional poverty. The spiral of losing control of personal autonomy and becoming unable to cope with the demands of day-to-day life can be heightened if a person has physical and associated disabilities and experiences high-risk factors in their relationships with 'significant others' or becomes excluded and isolated from the patterns of living which many people take for granted.

Definitions of what constitutes abuse are widespread. Mervyn Eastman defines it as 'the systematic maltreatment, physical, emotional or financial abuse of a person made vulnerable due to disability or age' (1984: 47). This may take the form of physical assault, threatening behaviour, neglect and abandonment or sexual assault.

Protection and safeguarding from abuse, however, should perhaps not be about overprotecting or segregating people and denying vulnerable people the pleasures and freedoms of everyday life. It is interesting to look back in time over past generations, where disabled people experienced decades of incarceration in long-stay institutions and separation from society not due to crime or illness, but simply due to their disability. Protection appeared to be afforded mainly to those non-disabled people who perceived disability as a threat, in some way dangerous, or a drain on society and wanted a division between 'them and us' to be sustained. It could be argued that institutional abuse has created the biggest cause of injustice to vulnerable people over a lengthy period of history. As recently as 2006, investigations into bad practice across some nursing homes in Cornwall discovered that staff were administering enemas to all patients, as a matter of course, and on a regular basis. This typifies the nature of institutional abuse, sustained over many years, where individuals are denied personal dignity, choice and control and can be subjected to infringements of their personal human rights and become vulnerable due to imposed and rigid treatments and regimes. This can create professional dilemmas for staff tasked to protect service users from potential risk of abuse from others by depriving them of liberty through practice such as locking doors, set times for meals and getting people up in the morning.

Although cases of institutional abuse are still happening, they are declining and being overtaken by other types of abuse, which are gaining ground as increasing sources of concern. Discriminatory abuse has increased, due to the number of vulnerable disabled people living in the community and experiencing victimization by individuals or groups of people. One of a number of real-life scenarios which caught media attention and progressed through the criminal justice system to the High Court of Justice in May 2008 can be briefly detailed.

Scenario for reflection

The case refers to a married couple with learning and physical disabilities who lived in their own flat in Hounslow with their two young daughters. The family were befriended by a group of young men who started to use the family home as a base for meeting their friends, drinking and drug dealing. The couple were imprisoned in their own home, locked in the bathroom and physically, sexually and psychologically abused. The abuse continued for several months, although the family were well known by the police, education and social services.

This example of opportunist harassment and abuse of a family who became vulnerable due to their disability highlights the difficulties of having a number of services aware of the risks for the family, but who are not working together in the best interests of the individuals needing support. Poor communication across agencies, different professional perspectives, disjointed assessments and a patchy adult safeguarding legislative framework may all be factors leading to the poor outcomes for this family, who were able to fall through the net of support that should have been protected them.

Reflection on practice

In what ways could agencies and professionals supporting the family have worked together to minimize the risks to the family and prevented the abuse happening? How could the parents have been empowered to ask for help when the threat of harm became apparent to them?

You may have considered current practice ideas such as single assessments, key working and advocacy back-up for the family. Local community capacity-building ideas, such as the use of volunteers to look out for vulnerable members of the community, could have helped to flag up the issues before the situation escalated.

This is a stark and disturbing example of a contemporary incident of abuse of disabled people which is a rare but frightening reminder of the risks to vulnerable people in ordinary society. This needs to be set in context with the experiences of many disabled people living in the UK who may experience lower levels of misfortune and hardship which could escalate towards harm and the potential for abuse. Research into the need for disabled refugees and asylum seekers to access social services and welfare benefits (Roberts and Harris 2002) has identified that, in many cases, people were not receiving the support needed to enable independent living. The issues experienced by many of the people interviewed included barriers created by English being the second language, a lack of awareness of individual linguistic needs and the overlooking of cultural and impairment needs. One case illustrating many of these points refers to a 42-year-old male asylum seeker with a visual impairment, diabetes and kidney failure, who described his experiences in this personal account:

> They called a car and they sent me here to live. The council gave the address to the mini cab driver and they brought me here. They didn't tell me where I was going . . . nothing . . . They used

to give me the frozen food . . . ready meal, for six to eight months. After that it made me sick. I am still suffering now with that food . . . I am Muslim . . . I don't eat any meat. They sent me Halal food . . . they sent me enough for a month or 20 days and they put it in a freezer here and each day they gave me two packs . . . believe me, that made me sick.

(Roberts and Harris 2002: 17)

This personal experience of a person living in the UK with very different religious and cultural beliefs and a number of health issues reflects how limited and insensitive support has not recognized or valued the person in terms of their right to information and access to the medical, social and personal support to which they are entitled.

Reflection on practice

If this man had been referred to you as a professional worker, what plans would you consider putting in place, both as an initial and intensive support plan and also for ongoing assistance?

There may have been many issues reflected on here, for example, a person-centred self-assessment to identify the range of issues from the service user's perspective, ensuring that the emotional shock and trauma of cultural and environmental change are responded to. Also, setting up links with local services, which are culturally sensitive and can provide natural networks of support.

Alaszewski (1998, cited in Mantell and Scragg 2008) makes a clear link between the social construction of risk and issues of vulnerability. He argues that society's preoccupation with risk has become politically linked with the way that resources are rationed. The targeting and gate-keeping role of local authorities, where eligibility for support is heavily prioritized, may be resulting in people becoming vulnerable due to their dependence on social care services and the barriers within society not being removed. This would indicate that the social model of disability is hard to sustain and there may be conflicts with social work values. For example, practice experience with individuals with a learning and physical disability suggests that they require consistent and enabling support. However, on occasions, practitioners report that they are put under pressure by budget constraints to make a short-term placement, instead of more appropriate provision because of the perceived cost of a package that might support a person to become more independent in the community.

Funding for a required support plan can be achieved through an emphasis on risk but this can also compromise practice that should be empowering. Tanner (1997: 451) found that to prove a person's eligibility, practitioners were 'obliged to stress the magnitude of their problems'.

The tension, therefore, between the reality of the resource rationing focus of service delivery and the philosophy of personalization and individual autonomy, appears to be having a negative impact on some disabled people who become too vulnerable due to poor or inadequate support to maintain a good standard of life within their community. This could be seen as a factor in the way that individuals can slip towards coping with increasing risks leading to harm and the potential to become abused.

Scenario for reflection

Elizabeth Mosely is a disabled activist who comes from a Christian background in Australia. Her powerful story relates to the spiritual strength she found in her religion and the marginalization she experienced as a newly disabled person. Mosely describes how her worship became a solitary and confining experience, as she was frequently unable to engage in the community church activities due to her physical disability. As a wheelchair user, she is often unable to fully access places of worship and finds herself behind pillars and pews if she is able to access the building. As an activist, she campaigns for herself and for other disabled people and gives examples of the oppression and exclusion that needs to be challenged: 'I have not lost my spirituality, simply my ability to walk . . . the very process of ageing with a disability causes an ever increasing number of problems with access for a regrettably large number of people. Their faith has not diminished, only their mobility' (Mosely 2004: 118–19).

The importance of spirituality as a central and human essence contributing to individual well-being has become increasingly significant as a factor in contemporary society. This may be particularly relevant where people have become estranged or isolated from their families and cultural networks. The progression of personalized ways to empower disabled people to articulate their needs and to express their preferences and choices which is central to modern-day social work seems to be in harmony with increased holistic and spiritual awareness. The emphasis on materialist and consumer access to rationed resources may well have created the human impetus to believe in spirituality as an agent of social change to recognize individuality and value difference.

A further contributing factor to the number of disabled people who are at risk of abuse may be the increase in the number of people who are directly involved in the care and support of disabled people. Carers are increasing; there are six million carers in the UK. An extract from the Department of Health White Paper (2006: 24–5) states: 'It is an interesting fact that if all unpaid carers were funded for the care provided, this would cost the government more than the entire cost of the National Health service'. The caring relationship between a vulnerable adult and their main carer has been explored over the years and has recently been challenged as a socially constructed interdependence, which could be oppressive due to the unequal relationship between the person dependent on care and the care giver. Kittay (1999) refers to the 'burden of care' and the power imbalance intrinsic in the relationship. Kittay makes a distinction between the justification of an unequal power relationship between a carer and a dependent adult and, when this becomes domination, an illegitimate exercise of power which can lead to abuse and deprivation of liberty and freedom of choice. It could be argued that the increasing pressure put upon carers due to influences such as the personalization agenda and increasing financial, social and psychological constraints experienced in daily life could be taking its toll and adding to the factors leading to the abuse of disabled people. Other important factors, such as the demographic increase in older, frailer people and those with dementia has also contributed to an increase in the number of older carers who may also be experiencing high levels of mental health issues such as anxiety, stress and depression.

There are also important gender-related issues bound up with the caring role for many disabled people. Feminist writers and activists have researched socially constructed ideas about women's role in society and the cycle of caring that prevails across generations, where women are often perceived to be the natural choice for caring for vulnerable partners or relatives. Millar and Glendinning (1989) also make the link between gender and poverty and the connection between poverty and need for social work help. The 'feminization of poverty' theory underlines the linkages between gender, oppression and social work.

Scenarios for reflection

Two cases receiving much public interest at the time of writing were both featured in the *Independent* newspaper (26 January 2010). Both cases refer to mothers who have cared for their disabled adult son/daughter and have ended their child's life to relieve them of their ongoing debilitating illnesses. Bridget Gilderdale supported her daughter's decision to end her own life by giving her morphine and drugs. Her daughter had contracted the chronic fatigue illness known as ME 11 years previously and was left paralysed from the waist down, unable to eat or drink and fed through a tube. Her daughter had made a 'living will' and had openly contemplated her own suicide. Bridget Gilderdale was found 'not guilty' of murder and had already admitted aiding and abetting suicide, for which she was given a 12-month conditional discharge.

This case offers a dramatic contrast with that of Frances Inglis, who was sentenced to life imprisonment for killing her disabled son. Her son had suffered acute brain damage in 2007 and could not speak. Mrs Inglis was charged with murder rather than assisted suicide, as there was no evidence that her son intended to take his own life.

It could be argued that both mothers acted in the best interests of their seriously ill son/daughter for whom they had cared over a number of years. The main difference between the two cases appears to be the capacity of the individual being cared for to consent to their lives being ended. The impact of adult social care legislation, such as the Human Rights Act (1988) Article 2 'Rights to Life' and the Mental Capacity Act (2005) can inform and guide practice and help to protect and safeguard people from harm, although as illustrated by these two cases, this is a complex and difficult process.

Reflection on practice

There may be dilemmas in practice when supporting both a service user and a carer and ensuring that the assessment process takes account of any conflicting views and priorities. An example would be a referral to visit a young disabled person living at home with her carer when the disabled person is planning to move into supported housing. The carer is unhappy with this plan and is concerned about the risks attached to increased independence. How could the tensions be explored in a professional and holistic way?

You may have considered both the self-assessment and the carer's assessment to gain both perspectives, a person-centred risk-taking assessment which clearly identifies both the risk and the gains attached to the risk taking and the right level of support required to ensure that changes are as positive and beneficial as possible to both the user and carer.

Positive responses to the vulnerability of disabled people to abuse

Many of the positive developments promoting adult disability and emphasizing the potential to counteract negative messages (such as the depicted images of disability held widely by society and the inherent difficulties of coping with impairment) have been made by disabled people themselves. Thompson (2003) suggests that, where there is a dominant ideology representing and reinforcing the position of powerful groups in society, there will also be countervailing ideologies. Such opposing ideologies can be seen to undermine the power domination of particular groups. The Disabled People's Movement recognizes that oppression emerging from prejudice and discrimination is a human creation, layered across personal, cultural and structural levels of society. The ideological belief that disabled people are a homogeneous group would be denying the complex impact of oppression across marginalized individuals, who may be black, gay, single parents and have one or more disabilities.

The BCODP (British Council of Organizations of Disabled People) is an affiliation of organizations representing disabled people, which steadily developed strength in the 1970s. Michael Oliver (1995) refers to the 'hierarchy of disabilities' and the preponderance of wheelchair users in positions of leadership, as compared to the representation from people with learning disabilities. Oliver makes the point that equality within the disability movement will only be truly achieved when people with learning disabilities are given positions of power and influence within the movement: 'One of the things we have to look at and be confident about is the reality of why most leaders in the disability movement are wheelchair users. It is very important that the movement has representation from every one of the major impairments'.

Learning point

A campaign spearheaded by the Leonard Cheshire Foundation has found an inspiring way to promote the experiences of young, physically disabled people in everyday life. By creating a series of animated films called *Creature Discomforts* designed and produced by the well-known film animators of *Creature Comforts*, humour and irony have been used as a medium to get messages across about the social and emotional poverty and oppression often experienced by young disabled people.

One of the characters portrayed in the film is a young black man who had a serious road traffic accident causing him to lose an arm and as a result of spine damage has become dependent on using a wheelchair. Due to his determination and personal resilience he was able to set himself up in his own home business making Caribbean food. In his words, 'people see us as a huge burden on the state but we can make things happen'.

The film portrays several young physically disabled people who are able to advocate for themselves to challenge the low expectations of society and to question the ideas and attitudes about disability which often deny the 'wholeness' of life taken for granted by non-disabled people. Another character in the film who has cerebral palsy and is a wheelchair user explains how disabled people can fear rejection and isolate themselves from people who don't have a disability. This person was able to promote her message by speaking up about her own personal relationship with a non-disabled man and how perceived barriers were reduced due to their determination to live an ordinary life and help to change the fundamental interactions with other human beings.

Reflection on practice

Disabled people can be proactive in advocating on behalf of people with disabilities and project positive messages which help to alter preconceptions about dependency and disempowerment. Consider some practical examples of disabled people you know who are active role models for the disabled movement.

You will have come up with your own examples, but three that spring to my mind are:

- a physically disabled person who has set up his own training consultancy to lecture to groups of students about discrimination and anti-oppressive practices;
- a physically and sensory disabled person who is employed with a housing development company to design homes which are fully accessible for disabled people;
- a group of disabled people who have set up a peer brokerage company to support other disabled people with their direct payments.

The diversity and heterogeneity within adult disability implies that there are not only differences due to gender, ethnicity, age and class but also social and financial differences. Norman (1985) suggests that older people with a disability may experience 'triple jeopardy', which means that age, cultural and racial discrimination and lack of access to health, housing and social services are major problems for many older people from ethnic minorities. (This will be explored in more detail in Chapter 8 where consideration will be given to the risks of harm and abuse for the older person).

Personalized responses to services have a vital role in combating the disabling impact of multiple disadvantage for individuals and there are positive examples of where support can be tailored to individual need and personal situations. Research has identified that black and minority ethnic people are considerably underrepresented among direct payment users, despite the potential of individual budgets to deliver a more culturally responsive service. (Butt et al. 2000). However, where this has been available, it has been welcomed. Research from the Joseph Rowntree Foundation (Clark et al. 2004) found that older Somali women with disabilities were able to secure culturally sensitive services through direct payments, where statutory agencies were not able to provide them with Somali-speaking care assistants. Having someone who can speak the same language was found to be crucial in enabling the Somali women to be in control and determine what was done for them.

When reflecting on established terminology and definitions which are then widely agreed and followed, it is possible to understand how value-loaded terms such as 'vulnerability' can lead to rigid practices and policies which are unhelpful to disabled people. Research which challenges accepted beliefs about disability and vulnerability is widening the horizons of thinking and introducing empowering and interesting ideas. Barbara Fawcett (2006) wrote an article in the journal of *International Social Work* which questions certainties in social work. The *'No Secrets'* (DoH 2000) definition of a vulnerable adult emphasizes the perceived weaknesses of individuals, rather than strengths. Fawcett argues that this implies dependency, passivity and the need for assistance, rather than the potential for autonomy and self-determination. The perceived helplessness of individuals who may be disempowered by the system of assessment and the need to seek help may weaken the capacity of individuals to demonstrate their capacity to cope and retain independence. Are more people becoming labelled as vulnerable as definitions of what constitutes disability widen? Perhaps it is more honest to advocate for a wider acceptance of vulnerability as potentially affecting anyone who may experience social exclusion, loss and crisis at some stage in their life?

Scenario for reflection

You are visiting an older couple, who are both aged 85, in their home. The man has chronic arthritis and the woman has sight impairment and diabetes.

> In what ways can risks be reduced to encourage inclusion and enable the couple to remain safely in their own home?
>
> You may have considered focusing on each person's strengths and ways to minimize risk in the least invasive way in order to enable the couple to help each other. Tele-care can be helpful as a back-up to provide support such as regular phone calls, monitoring of aids and adaptations and internet ordering.

Person-centred approaches, when supporting disabled people, can certainly be helpful in preventing vulnerability to harm and potential abuse and are central to the social work 'tool kit' of good practice-based skills and knowledge. Titterton (2005) makes a clear link between identified need and actual risks in day-to-day life and advocates person-centred risk taking as an important step towards breaking barriers and empowering people to feel less vulnerable and more in control of their lives. Titterton sees communication as at the heart of good personalized risk assessment, which should encompass 'physical, psychological, and emotional well being, rights and responsibilities, abilities and disabilities, choices and opportunities and involve the individual and their family carers' (2005: 82). This holistic approach appears to be vital in ensuring that the direct link between risk, need and vulnerability does not further disable individuals who may experience a rationing of resources and support due to narrow 'safety first' assessment processes.

Kemshall (2002) warns that it is potentially oppressive to assume that a person is 'vulnerable' merely because they appear to be in need of social care services. This author refers to the social construction of risk and the apparent contradictions with the principles of the social model of disability.

Physically disabled people may have visible and invisible impairments and have experienced negativity and oppression in their lives, which may collectively result in their vulnerability. The government mandated National Equality Panel (2010) identifies a wider disparity between the wealthy and less wealthy now than in the last 40 years. The link between unequal societies and low social mobility has impacted on physically disabled people, as it has with other minority groups in the UK, to create challenges and low expectations by others about what can be achieved. Some examples of positive responses to challenging exclusion and threats of harm and abuse have been included to redress the balance and demonstrate how positive social policy, advocacy and person-centred responses to supporting people can offer positive alternatives. Social models of disability are important vehicles in deconstructing the barriers created over time which can exclude, oppress and marginalize people who are perceived as different because of a physical disability. Hopefully this chapter has stimulated interest and reinforced the collective responsibility we share in recognizing and responding to discrimination and the need to protect people from harm. As expressed by the *Creature Discomforts* spokesperson for the Leonard Cheshire Foundation, 'we can try to change society's view of physically disabled people by lecturing them, hectoring them, by regulation, or by changing the fundamental ways we interact with other human beings' (personal communication).

Note

1   A key source of information on this troubled historical period is the Centre for Holocaust and Genocide Studies at the University of Minnesota in Minneapolis, USA (www.chgs.umn.edu).

Chapter summary

The chapter has explored many factors in contemporary society which are relevant to disabled people, and has particularly highlighted the ways that disability can make adults vulnerable to risks of harm and abuse. Chapter themes can be summarized as follows:

- reflection on the historical, social and political context of disability helps us to highlight the barriers still experienced by individuals in contemporary society;
- illustration through case studies and reflective exercises helps us to understand the ways that disabled people can be marginalized and risks develop into harm and abuse;
- we have seen the importance of recognizing diversity of disability, often encompassing many layers, due to multiple impairments and links with eligibility to assessment and intervention;
- the chapter has made reference to approaches which challenge discrimination and abuse, and which promote inclusion by recognizing the strengths of individuals perceived to be vulnerable by society.

References

Brown, K. (2010) *Vulnerable Adults and Community Care*. Exeter: Learning Matters.

Butt, J., Bignall, T. and Stone, E. (eds) (2000) *Directing Support: Report from a Workshop on Direct Payments and Black and Minority Ethnic Disabled People*. York: Joseph Rowntree Foundation.

Cambridge, P. (2007) *In Safe Hands, Protecting People with Learning Disabilities from Abuse*. Brighton: Pavilion.

Cambridge, P. and Carnaby, S. (2005) *Person Centred Planning and Care Management with People with Learning Disabilities.* London: Jessica Kingsley.

Campbell, J. and Oliver, M. (1995) *Disability Politics.* London: Routledge.

Clark, H., Dyer, S. and Horwood, J. (1988) *That Bit of Help: The High Value of Low Level Preventative Services for Older People.* Bristol/York: The Policy Press/Joseph Rowntree Foundation.

Clark, H., Gough, H. and MacFarlane, A. (2004) *Making Direct Payments Work for Older People.* York: Joseph Rowntree Foundation.

Commission for Social Care Inspection and Commission for Healthcare Audit and Inspection (2006) *Joint Inspection into the Provision of Services for People with Learning Disabilities at Cornwall Partnership NHS* Trust. London: Commission for Healthcare Audit and Inspection.

Danaher, G. (2000) *Understanding Foucault.* London: Sage.

Davis, L. (1997) *The Disability Studies.* London: Routledge.

Department for Constitutional Affairs (2007) *The Mental Capacity Act Code of Practice.* London: TSO.

Department of Health (DoH) (2000) *'No Secrets': Guidance on Developing and Implementing Multi-Agency Protection of Vulnerable Adults.* London: TSO.

Department of Health (DoH) (2002) *Fair Access to Care Services: Eligibility Criteria for Adult Social Care.* London: TSO.

Department of Health (DoH) (2006) White Paper: *Our Health, Our Care, Our Say, and Launch of a New Deal for Carers.* London: TSO.

Department of Health (DoH) (2007) *Putting People First: A Shared Vision and Commitment to the Transformation of Adult Social Care.* London: Department of Health.

Eastman, M. (1984) *Old Age Abuse.* Mitcham: Age Concern.

Fawcett, B. (2006) Vulnerability: questioning the certainties in social work and health, *International Social Work*, 52(4): 473–84.

Ferrero, G. (1911) *Criminal Man.* New York: Knickerbocker Press.

Fine, M. and Glendinning, C. (2005) Dependence, independence or inter-dependence? Re-visiting the concepts of 'care' and 'dependency', *Ageing and Society* 25, 601–21.

Galpin, D. and Bates, N. (2009) *Social Work Practice with Adults.* Exeter: Learning Matters.

Hales, G. (1996) *Beyond Disability.* Buckingham: Open University Press.

IBSEN (2008) *The National Evaluation of the Individual Budgets Pilot Programme* (research findings). York: Social Policy Research Unit.

Kemshall, H. (2002) *Risk, Social Policy and Welfare.* Buckingham: Open University Press.

Kittay, E. (1999) *Love's Labour: Essays on Women, Equality and Dependency.* London: Routledge.

Leonard Cheshire Disability (2009) *Creature Discomforts.* Disability Campaign. Available at: www.creaturediscomforts.org.

Lombroso, C. (1911) Cited in Ferrero, G., *Criminal Man*. New York: Knickerbocker Press.

Mantell, A. (2009) *Social Work Skills with Adults*. Exeter: Learning Matters.

Mantell, A. and Scragg, T. (2008) *Safeguarding Adults in Social Work*. Exeter: Learning Matters.

Matthews, I. (2009) *Social Work and Spirituality*. Exeter: Learning Matters.

Millar, J. and Glendinning, C. (1989) 'Gender and Poverty', *Journal of Social Policy* 18: 363–81.

Mosely, E. (2004) Solitary confinement in the forgotten ministry. In C. Newell and A. Calder (eds) *Voices in Disability and Spirituality from the Land Down Under: Outback to Outfront*. Binghampton, NY: Haworth Press.

National Equality Panel (2010) *An Anatomy of Economic Inequality in the UK: Report of the National Equality Panel*. Available at: www.equalities.gov.uk/national_equality_panel/publications.aspx.

Norman, A. (1985) *Triple Jeopardy: Growing Old in Second Homeland*. London: Centre for Policy on Ageing.

Oliver, M. (1996) *Understanding Disability: From Theory to Practice*. Basingstoke: Macmillan.

Oliver, M. and Barnes, C. (1998) *Disabled People and Social Policy*. London: Longman.

Pater, J.E. (1981) *The Making of the National Health Service*. London: Kings Fund.

Roberts, K. and Harris, J. (2002) *Disabled People in Refugee and Asylum Seeking Communities*. Oxford: Policy Press and the Joseph Rowntree Foundation.

Sibley, D. (1995) *Geographies of Exclusion*. London: Routledge.

Swain, J., Finklestein, V., French, S. and Oliver, M. (1996) *Disabling Barriers: Enabling Environments*. London: Sage.

Tanner, D. (1997) Eligibility and comparative need. In D. Galpin and N. Bates (eds) *Social Work Practice with Adults*. Exeter: Learning Matters.

Thompson, N. (2003) *Anti-discriminatory Practice*. Basingstoke: Macmillan.

Titterton, M. (2005) *Risk and Risk Taking in Health and Social Welfare*. London: Jessica Kingsley.

Williams, P. (2006) *Social Work with People with Learning Disabilities*. Exeter: Learning Matters.

Other sources

Case Notes for the Hounslow case (case no. HQ03X03456) Royal Courts of Justice, London.

The National Evaluation of the Individual Budgets Pilot Programme, www.york.ac.uk/spru.

Creature Discomforts 2. Leonard Cheshire Disability's Campaign, www.CreatureDiscomforts.org, 2008.

3   Sensory impairments

Melanie Parris

Sensory impairments represent a significant domain of risk among adults. While some sensory impairments are present from birth, others are acquired during the life-cycle, with the result that an adult must make the difficult accommodation to impairment, combating not only the physical difficulty itself but the stigma, discrimination and oppressive treatment associated with much impairment. The current chapter takes the case study of a specific 'hidden impairment' – acquired hearing loss – as a forum for exploring the challenges faced by sensorily impaired adults. We will consider some of the consequences of acquiring a sensory impairment such as deafness in adulthood, the discrimination often experienced and the risks which can ensue. The latter part of the chapter examines ways in which professionals can work in partnership with service users to minimize risks, intervening on a number of levels, building on service users' strengths and utilizing a range of resources and services.

Learning objectives

Readers of this chapter will be able to:

- understand the discrimination and stigma faced by adults with a 'hidden impairment' such as acquired hearing loss;
- describe the key facts about acquired hearing loss;
- explain the effects of acquired hearing loss in increasing the likelihood of risk and social exclusion;
- identify challenges for practice when working with people with hidden impairments;
- employ effective communication strategies when working with people with hidden impairments;
- identify and utilize resources and services to promote social inclusion, reduce risks and enhance quality of life.

Why hidden impairments should concern professionals

The concept of hidden impairments encompasses a wide range of conditions, which are not visible. These include, for example, specific learning disabilities such as dyslexia and dyspraxia, or other conditions such as speech and language difficulties, and medical conditions such as heart disease, lupus, diabetes, ME, or mental health conditions, Crohn's disease and so on. The Equality Act 2010 defines a disabled person as 'someone who has a physical or mental impairment that has substantial and long-term adverse effect on the person's ability to carry out normal day-to-day activities', making no overt distinction between the treatment of individuals with visible and 'hidden' impairments.

It is likely that when asked to picture a disabled person, a large proportion of respondents would think of a wheelchair user, and yet wheelchair users form a minority of the total population of disabled people in the UK; there are significant numbers of people with non-visible impairments, for example nearly two million people in the UK have a visual impairment (Access Economics 2008).

Unlike people with more visible impairments, people with hidden impairments face the dilemma of whether to disclose or attempt to avoid disability discrimination by trying to 'pass' as non-disabled. For example, the report 'From Compliance to Culture Change' commissioned by NIACE in 2008 to look at disabled staff in the lifelong learning sector, found that although 1 in 5 staff had an impairment, only 1 in 25 felt able to disclose it (Commission for Disabled Staff in Lifelong Learning 2008).

It may be tempting to try to avoid possible discrimination and stigma by maintaining a façade of 'normality' (French 2004). However, adopting this strategy means missing out on necessary reasonable adjustments and support, and may incur a cost for the individual in terms of effort, energy expended and pain incurred. In these circumstances tension can be caused by the need to make complex judgements about the costs vs benefits of disclosing. For example, in a job interview is it better to disclose a hearing impairment and request support, which may lead to unconscious prejudice or assumptions about competence, or is it more beneficial to hide one's deafness and risk miscommunication and failure? The anxiety caused by such dilemmas exacerbates what is already a stressful situation.

When impairment is not visible it is more likely to be denied or questioned by other people, and that judgements are made on the basis of prejudice, for example that a deaf person can 'hear when they want to' or that a person using a disabled parking space is not entitled to so do. These questions deny the efforts made to carry out daily activities, which people without a disability take for granted. Having a hidden impairment for many people means being the focus of unwanted attention and scrutiny and being forced to explain and justify matters which are intensely personal.

Models of disability

The social model of disability recognizes the impact of society and the wider environment in creating and perpetuating disability and disadvantage through structural factors, including lack of appropriate services and attitudinal barriers, and by pathologizing people with impairments. This model of disability moves the focus of attention away from the individual and examines the way in which the wider environment places restrictions on them (Oliver and Sapey 2006). Such a view contrasts with the medical model of disability, where the 'problem' or 'deficiency' is located within the disabled person, who is the object of treatment and intervention to enable them to better fit into society. The social model of disability promotes the view that society should change to better meet the needs of disabled people rather than disabled people changing to meet the requirements of society. Within the overarching framework of the social model, it is possible also to acknowledge the personal and psychological effects of impairment, which in the case of hearing loss can be significant.

Deafness as an impairment

There are significant debates around whether D/deafness does indeed constitute an impairment (see e.g. Corker 2002). Members of the Deaf community might well dispute that deaf people are disabled, perceiving D/deafness to be a cultural issue, and seeing themselves as part of a cultural minority rather than the wider disabled population, or movement. By contrast, people who have an acquired or partial loss would be more likely to identify themselves as being disabled, particularly if they lose their hearing in adulthood, having previously identified themselves as hearing. This chapter supports the latter view and looks at the effects of impairment across a range of levels from the personal to the wider social, environmental and ultimately political domains.

Hearing loss as a hidden impairment

As explained earlier, this chapter considers acquired hearing loss as a case study to illustrate some of the many issues concerned with hidden impairments. Acquired hearing loss is an under-researched subject even within the field of Deaf Studies. However, this chapter argues that it is crucial for professionals to be informed about this type of hearing impairment for a number of reasons.

First, acquired hearing loss has a high prevalence and intersects with other individual and structural factors to increase risk. Therefore it is likely that any professional working with adults will encounter people with acquired hearing loss either knowingly or unknowingly. Second, the impact of acquired hearing loss is significant and may be compounded by the fact that people with an acquired hearing loss often do not acknowledge or admit that their hearing has declined. Third, lack of knowledge and awareness can lead to ineffective practice with risks to service users going unchallenged. Finally, awareness underpins effective practice with service users and can promote positive outcomes.

Acquired hearing loss shares commonalities with other hidden impairments. For example, denial of hearing loss is prevalent and in part due to stigma which is manifested through stereotyping and humour directed against D/deaf people. While terms such as 'deaf and dumb' are no longer as commonly used, and are considered offensive, it is still considered acceptable, for example, to talk about arguments 'falling on deaf ears', a phrase commonly used in the media and everyday conversation.

The use of prevailing myths is another mechanism for denial of the impact of hearing loss (Royal National Institute for Deaf People (RNID) 2010). There are two key myths relating to deafness: that lipreading is a fairly straightforward way to facilitate communication and that hearing aids restore hearing in the same way that glasses restore sight. In fact, lipreading is not an exact science and only a small proportion of words can be understood by a skilled lipreader. There are a variety of reasons for this: some speakers are easier than others to follow because of the shape of their mouths, clarity of speech, and the familiarity of their accent. It is easier to recognize familiar words, which has implications for service users whose first language is not English. The speed at which people speak is also a factor and some words are extremely difficult, if not impossible, to lipread or look identical to the lipreader. Contrary to the second myth, hearing aids do not restore full hearing for people with sensorineural deafness. They only amplify sounds which can be heard using residual hearing, and despite recent advances in hearing aid technology and the advent of digital aids, background noise and the altered quality and nature of the sounds heard through the aid are often problematic for wearers. In some areas there are currently lengthy waiting times for NHS aids which can be as long as two years. Hearing aids are expensive and can cost several thousand pounds if purchased privately.

Facts about hearing loss

According to Action on Hearing Loss (formerly known as the Royal National Institute for Deaf People) It is estimated that approximately nine million people in the UK have some degree of hearing loss, which equates to 1 in 7 of the population, and the large majority of these will have an acquired loss, having been born fully hearing, and subsequently losing a proportion of their hearing in adulthood. Hearing loss significantly increases with age and is estimated to affect 41.7 per cent of people over the age of 50, and 71 per cent of those over the age of 70. In contrast there are estimated to be around 20,000 children and young people from birth to 15 years who have a moderate to profound hearing loss (RNID 2010). The causes of loss are varied and include genetic predisposition, trauma, viral infections, the side effects of some drugs/medication, and exposure to noise.

Hearing impairment is linked with other impairments, for example with sight loss in Usher's Syndrome, and with Down's syndrome and other learning disabilities. There is anecdotal evidence that certain ethnic groups, for example the Romany, Gypsy and Traveller community, and South East Asian communities in the UK, experience a heightened prevalence of hearing loss. This requires professionals to be aware of the way in which culture and other structural factors intersect with D/deafness to create disadvantage.

Scenario for reflection

Imagine you are working with Kojo, an asylum seeker, who has limited spoken English and a hearing impairment. What issues would you need to be aware of? What information might you need in order to work effectively in partnership with Kojo?

There are two major types of hearing loss: conductive and sensorineural deafness. Sensorineural deafness is far more prevalent and likely to affect adults. It is caused by damage to the hair cells in the inner ear which transmit sound waves to the brain and accounts for most age-related deafness. This form of hearing impairment is currently irreversible, as the damaged cells cannot be repaired or replaced. The effect is usually a loss of the high frequencies because the hair cells which transmit these sounds are more fragile and more susceptible to damage. This means that a person with high-frequency loss will hear the vowels rather than the consonants of speech and may rely on lipreading to make sense of speech.

The other less common form of deafness is conductive deafness where there is some form of damage to the mechanism by which sound is conducted through the ear, for example damage to the bones within the ear. This type of deafness may often be surgically corrected, and people with conductive deafness can usually obtain greater benefit from hearing aids than those with sensorineural loss.

The effects of acquired hearing loss

On a personal level the effects of loss of hearing in adulthood will vary from individual to individual depending not only on the type and severity of the loss, but also on the individual's resilience and the influence of structural factors such as culture, social class, and formal and informal support networks. Unlike people who are culturally Deaf, people who are born hearing and become deafened may experience a sense of being left in a limbo, no longer part of the hearing world but not part of the Deaf community either. People with acquired hearing loss move into uncharted territory, and may be forced to confront their own prejudices about deafness and deaf people. The acquisition of hearing loss therefore raises issues around the way in which impairment is viewed as an individual failing (Hogan 2001).

The significant psychological effects of becoming deaf should not be underestimated. As one book puts it, 'becoming deafened in adult life is a life changing event with profound consequences. The emotional impact is always strong. People commonly describe anger, helplessness, frustration and deep despair. Often they feel overwhelmingly isolated and lonely. Rates of depression amongst newly deafened people are high' (Hearing Concern/ LINK 2008–9: 10). Although referring to people who have become severely deaf, the statement may also apply to people with a lesser degree of acquired hearing loss.

Hearing loss can be accompanied by tinnitus, a condition where sounds are heard, sometimes referred to as 'head noises'. The sounds may take many different forms and fluctuate in severity and frequency, interfering with the ability to hear speech and resulting in anxiety. Although it is not entirely clear what causes tinnitus, it is thought that it is exacerbated and possibly caused by stress or exposure to loud noise, head injuries or as a result of hearing loss (Butler 2004). Tinnitus is also present in Menieres Disease which is linked with disturbance to the organ of balance in the inner ear and usually occurs in mid life. In addition to loss of hearing, the effects include vertigo, loss of balance and extreme nausea, and attacks can last for periods of up to several days. Menieres Disease usually commences in mid life after the age of 30 and before the age of 60. John's narrative gives some insight into the felt experience of this condition.

Scenario for reflection: John's experience

One morning I was struck by a severe attack of vertigo. I lay on the floor unable to move. The sensation of rotation was so severe that I was effectively blinded, every time I looked up the room was spinning so fast that I vomited violently; in addition I lost control of both my bladder and bowels. As a result, I received treatment and medication which alleviated but not cured the condition.

The onset of Menieres has had a huge impact on my life. I can go for several months in between attacks but although the severity and frequency of the condition has diminished, I never know when an attack could start. I would describe the biggest effect as living with constant fear. Like other people with Menieres, I am extremely anxious about going out in public in case a vertigo attack strikes. My hearing has also been affected and I struggle in social situations.

The impact of Menieres has been dramatic and I literally lost everything overnight, my career, and the ability to live the life I had before the attacks started; some of my friends lost patience and gave up on me as I was unable to go out and socialize.

Fortunately I was helped by a number of people; my ENT Consultant was enormously supportive and empathic and referred me for a hearing aid which has helped me not only to hear more effectively, but also to maintain my balance. An excellent hearing therapist helped in a number of ways, by enabling me to adapt to using the hearing aid and through rebalancing exercises. The Menieres Society has been a useful source of information, and has enabled me to network with others with the condition for peer support.

I was also very fortunate in being referred to a voluntary day service for people with mental health needs which gave me a positive focus to my life and through this I became involved in working with a university which restored my sense of self-esteem. The response from student social workers to my teaching has been amazing and very positive. Although Menieres Disease is a constant presence, I have slowly been able to rebuild my life and am now a service user consultant for a number of universities.

John's experience of hearing loss was made particularly traumatic by the associated severe attacks of vertigo, but his narrative encapsulates some common themes linked with hearing loss. These include the sense of ever present fear and anxiety about social and public situations, compounded by popular misconceptions and lack of knowledge, the loss of employment and financial security, replaced by dependence on benefits, and the risk of marginalization and social exclusion.

Risks associated with loss of hearing

There are several risks associated with loss of hearing:

- loss of environmental sounds: heightened risk of missing warning and orienting sounds, enhanced risk of accidents and crime;
- psychological effects: internalized oppression, low self-esteem, anxiety, depression, risk of suicide, social withdrawal leading to risk of abuse and exploitation;
- social relationships: relationship breakdown, social isolation, stigmatization, social exclusion;
- professional relationships: enhanced power imbalance, miscommunication, failure to develop rapport, flawed assessments and plans/ service provision;
- structural effects: heightened risk of unemployment, educational underachievement, financial hardship and difficulties in accessing benefits and services.

Acquired hearing loss may lead to a number of areas of risk resulting from loss of ability to hear sounds. Val Tait discusses the risks associated with loss of three categories of sounds: warning, environmental and social sounds (Tait 2007). Risks arising from loss of warning sounds include greater risk of physical harm. Although many deaf people become accustomed to relying on their sight rather than hearing when out in the community, they will be at danger from things which are outside their range of vision. A fairly common example is that of cyclists using the pavement approaching from behind, or lorries reversing relying on the reversing warning to alert pedestrians.

Using public transport can be anxiety provoking and challenging, as many warning announcements and information about platform changes are made via public address systems even when there are visual displays available. Any system which relies on people using their hearing including help points at train stations will be inaccessible to many deaf people.

Environmental sounds include the range of everyday sounds which keep people in contact with the environment and their surroundings, and which provide a sense of orientation and security. These could include the noise of traffic, or sounds of floorboards creaking, or the radio playing in another room. The loss of these sounds can lead to disorientation and anxiety, together with a sense of being distanced from the surrounding environment.

Loss of social sounds, and also the difficulties associated with hearing in noisy environments may lead to social isolation, loss of self-esteem, anxiety and depression, leaving people isolated at risk of abuse:

> Being severely deaf is very stressful, I feel isolated especially in groups – it is hard to keep up with the conversation. I get anxious about social situations and am on medication for that and depression

and stress. I avoid speaking to people if I think I won't be able to hear. I know if I could hear I would be much more outgoing.

(Helen)

As Helen articulates, loss of hearing means that communication and interaction with other people become more challenging and stressful. Understanding conversation requires effort, concentration and energy; it becomes time consuming because it is no longer possible to listen and engage in other activities at the same time. Acquired deafness requires other people in the family and social network to adapt their communication strategies, and this may result in difficulties within the relationship, although conversely it may strengthen them (Morgan-Jones 2001).

In addition to the risks outlined above, potentially serious risks to service users arise in interactions with professionals. Misdiagnosis and inaccurate assessments can occur if the practitioner is not communicating effectively and the service user misunderstands or mishears as a consequence. Loss of hearing can further exacerbate power differentials inherent in the service user–professional dynamic and the service user may not feel able to challenge a practitioner to communicate in a more helpful manner, by looking at them when they speak rather than reading their notes, or by moving to sit where the light falls on their face to facilitate lipreading.

Miscommunication can have profound implications in assessments of mental capacity, not only during the assessment process itself where miscommunication may occur, but also indirectly, given that hearing loss excludes people from the possibility of acquiring information and keeping up to date with current affairs through overhearing conversations or listening to the radio, and when hearing loss leads to social withdrawal and social exclusion.

Scenario for reflection

Peggy Smith is an 85-year-old widow who lives alone in a privately owned bungalow. Her daughter Mary is concerned because she feels that Peggy is becoming forgetful and confused. Several times recently she seemed to lose the thread of the conversation while talking on the phone to both Mary and her other daughter Liz. A recent optician's appointment was missed because of confusion over the time Peggy was to be collected. Peggy's neighbours, Arthur and Shirley, are upset because she ignored them when they shouted 'hello' over the fence.

You have been asked to carry out an assessment of Peggy. What would you need to be aware of to ensure that you gain an accurate picture of her strengths and any areas of need?

To conclude, major areas of risk for people with acquired hearing loss include: the impact of loss which can include low self-esteem, feelings of anger and frustration, loneliness, isolation, lowered quality of social life and effect on close relationships, employment and status, financial loss, anxiety/depression and risk of suicide. These may result in an enhanced risk of exploitation and abuse of all forms, physical, sexual, financial and emotional. Professional intervention may be affected by communication difficulties and miscommunication, but professionals have a responsibility to ensure that they use appropriate communication strategies in negotiation with the service user.

Strategies for empowering practice

As hearing loss impacts on people on a number of different levels, effective professional practice benefits from a systemic approach to the issues, working not only to empower individuals but to draw on resources in the community and harness the power of collective action, solidarity and political action/ lobbying.

John's narrative and accounts by other writers demonstrates that it is possible for people to move from a position of disempowerment to regain control and a sense of purpose through utilizing strategies for managing and adapting to the altered situation created by the onset of the impairment (Morgan-Jones 2001; Simmons 2005). John's experience demonstrates that professionals who are empathic, knowledgeable and skilled in working in partnership with deafened people can be instrumental in helping them to regain quality of life.

Empowering professional practice will include an open-minded awareness of the impact of acquired hearing loss and knowledge of appropriate communication strategies to ensure clear communication. In John's case he was able to benefit from technological solutions and the advice and support provided by voluntary sector organizations as well as peer support. Building on this support and his own resilience and skills, John is now playing a part in shaping the education of professional social workers through his work as a consultant at a number of universities.

The personal level

Skilled and empathic communication lies at the heart of work in the people professions, and in the field of social work communication is seen as essential (see for example Trevithick 2005; Lishman 2009; Moss 2009). Skilled communication has even greater significance for work with deaf service users, where miscommunication has potentially profound implications for assessments and interventions. In addition to the fundamental communication skills common to disciplines such as social work and counselling, there are specific communication strategies which enhance communication with people who have a hearing loss.

The basis of effective communication is to determine what the service user finds helpful, and to be adaptable and flexible in putting this into practice so that communication becomes a shared, negotiated and creative process. Respect for the service user should lie at the heart of professional interaction, though this is not always the case:

> A member of staff at my local audiology unit was very rude about me when I had my hearing aid out. She began complaining about me to a colleague. I had gone with a friend and she heard this woman moaning about me, and saying all these things in front of me, knowing full well that I couldn't hear.
>
> (Helen)

Communication strategies

The key to effective communication lies in building a relationship where the service user feels respected, valued and safe enough to indicate their communication needs, and not to be embarrassed about their deafness. Making sense of speech takes slightly longer for people who are lipreading, and appropriate time needs to be allowed. Awareness of body language is crucial; service users will soon pick up on signals that the professional is becoming impatient and may give rushed responses in an attempt to allow the interaction to move forward at the pace expected by the professional, rather than at a pace which allows them to process and make sense of information and respond appropriately. Service users also need to feel able to disclose when something has not been heard and needs to be clarified or repeated.

Other effective strategies include the following:

- Choose an appropriate, softly furnished environment with minimal background noise, for example, not near to a photocopier or busy office space. (Drawing the curtains round a hospital bed does not exclude background noise, neither does it ensure confidentiality.)
- Ensure that your lips are clearly visible and that there is good lighting on your face and not from behind, which throws the face into shadow, avoid sitting with your back to a window.
- Sit on the same level to aid lipreading, and not in very close proximity as the person lipreading will need to see your whole face and read your body language.

- Speak clearly without making exaggerated lip movements which can be perceived as patronizing, and make lipreading harder as the words are distorted.
- Rephrase rather than repeating words and phrases as there may be difficulty lipreading particular words or phrases.
- Give the service user a copy of the assessment form so that they can read what is being asked.
- If using an interpreter or supporter, always address the service user and look at them rather than the interpreter.
- Summarize and check that the key points of the conversation have been understood.

Scenario for reflection

Imagine you are working with Reg Lee who has recently been admitted to hospital with a chest infection. Reg has used a hearing aid for the past ten years. What communication strategies would you need to employ when interviewing Reg on the ward?

Legislation and support

At the time of writing some disabled people were feeling under attack from the government's drive to cut welfare spending and the specific attention which was being focused on people claiming disability benefits. Professionals can play a vital role in defending the rights of service users by providing knowledgeable support and advocacy on benefits issues, or being able to signpost to specialist advice services for disabled people.

The major legislation relating to disability is the Equality Act 2010 which has incorporated and harmonized existing legislation relating to areas of discrimination, including the Disability Discrimination Acts 1995 and 2005. Although legislation has led to some improvements in terms of equality for disabled people, as Harris and Bamford (2001) highlight, the road to equality and access to services is still an 'uphill' one for deaf people.

Employment

The Equality Act requires employers to make reasonable adjustments for disabled employees. Adapting the working environment to minimize background noise by providing a separate office or by providing specialist equipment, such as an amplified telephone, or the provision of deaf awareness training for colleagues would constitute reasonable adjustments under the Act, as would providing a parking space close to the entrance for a person with limited mobility.

Information about the Equality Act 2010 and examples of reasonable adjustments can be found on the website of the Equality and Human Rights Commission.

The Access to Work scheme accessed via Jobcentre Plus is designed to fund equipment and support services to enable disabled people to gain or remain in employment, where appropriate, after an initial assessment of need has been carried out. Examples of support include the provision of equipment or speech to text reporters or note takers who provide support at meetings. There are significant regional variations in the quality of support offered by Access to Work, and in the quality of assessment which may be carried out by private companies.

Education

The Equality Act 2010 places a responsibility on education providers to ensure that their provision is accessible to disabled students, and that disabled students are not discriminated against. Deaf and/or disabled students may be eligible, following assessment to qualify for a Disabled Students Allowance, to purchase support or equipment such as a radio microphone for use in lecture theatres and teaching rooms. Universities employ advisers who can offer support and guidance to disabled students. Ironically, D/deaf staff in higher education may fare less well than students. The NIACE Report referred to earlier (Commission for Disabled Staff in Lifelong Learning 2008) found widespread institutional discrimination against disabled employees in the Lifelong Learning Sector.

Welfare benefits

At the time of writing the government was in the process of revising the benefits paid to disabled people and had signalled its intention to end the Disability Living Allowance, which deaf people may be eligible for, replacing it with the Personal Independence Payment. Given current uncertainties over eligibility for disability benefits it is worth seeking benefit advice from disability law services, or voluntary organizations such as Action on Hearing Loss/RNID, which publishes information on benefits and services for deaf people.

There are a range of third-sector organizations for D/deaf and hearing impaired people, along with organizations of and for disabled people in general. These organizations tend to be relevant for specific sections of the D/deaf population, so for example the National Association for Deafened People addresses the needs of people who are deafened. Action on Hearing Loss, formerly known as the Royal National Institute for Deaf People, is the largest voluntary organization in the UK in relation to deafness; it campaigns on issues and provides a range of services and advice.

Other voluntary organizations include Hearing Concern/Link, formed from a merger of two existing organizations, one of which (Hearing Concern) was established to support partially hearing adults. The Link Centre was established in Eastbourne in 1972 to provide support for people with an acquired profound hearing loss; it runs intensive six-day residential courses for deafened people and family members and takes referrals from across the country. The cost of attending the courses may be met by the health authority. In addition to the large voluntary organizations there are a large number of local clubs, support groups and lipreading classes which offer the possibility of peer support, solidarity and collective action.

As well as deafness-specific organizations, general disability organizations both 'of' and 'for' disabled people can offer advice, support and links to other services. Professionals can play a valuable role by signposting service users to appropriate organizations, or by engaging in the campaigns run by organizations to improve services and challenge the stigma faced by people who have a hearing loss. Although legislation and services exist, it is by no means a straightforward matter for D/deaf people to gain access to their legal rights, and there are many challenges in this arena which will benefit from skilled professional support and advocacy. As professionals, we can play a role in enabling service users to gain the benefits and services to which they are entitled.

Principles of empowering practice summarized

- Be mindful of possible 'hidden impairments' such as hearing or sight loss in all interactions.
- Approach each situation prepared to learn from service users as experts about their lived experience.
- Develop a knowledge base about sensory impairments and other 'hidden impairments'.
- Create a safe environment for disclosure and discussion of issues.
- Listen to and value the service user's experience.
- Challenge assumptions and prejudicial attitudes towards deafness and other hidden impairments, both your own and others.

- Develop skills in communicating clearly and find out what helps the service user.
- Build on service users' strengths and employ creativity.
- Signpost service users to services, resources, peer support.
- Advocate for service users and challenge oppression.
- Be knowledgeable about the legislation and policy in relation to hidden impairments.
- Forge alliances and networks.

Chapter summary

- Hearing loss is a prevalent, misunderstood and hidden impairment, and professionals working with adults need to be aware of the possibility that whoever they work with may have a hearing loss or another hidden impairment.
- Deafened adults, and disabled people in general, face discrimination and disadvantage in all areas of life. Legislation exists to combat discrimination.
- The psychological aspects of hidden impairments and specifically hearing loss can be severe for some and should not be discounted. They include anxiety and depression which can lead to social withdrawal, impact on relationships and exacerbate risks of abuse and exploitation.
- The stigma faced by deaf and other disabled people leads to risks and service users may find valuable support in third-sector organizations, self-help groups and user-led organizations.
- Professionals can intervene to promote quality of life for service users in a number of areas, including employment, education and access to benefits and services.
- Specific communication skills and knowledge of what promotes effective communication are crucial for effective professional engagement.
- Principles of empowering practice are vital for effective professional intervention.

References

Access Economics (2008) *Future Sight Loss UK1: Economic Impact of Partial Sight and Blindness in the UK Adult Population.* London: RNIB.

Butler, S. (2004) *Hearing and Sight Loss: A Handbook for Professional Carers.* London: Age Concern England.

Commission for Disabled Staff in Lifelong Learning (2008) *From Compliance to Culture Change*. London: NIACE.

Corker, M. (2002) Deafness/disability: problematising notions of identity and culture. In S. Redell and N. Watson (eds) *Disability, Culture and Identity*. London: Pearson.

French, S. (2004) 'Can you see the rainbow': the roots of denial. In J. Swain et al. (eds) *Disabling Barriers: Enabling Environments*. London: Sage.

Harris, J. and Bamford, C. (2001) The uphill struggle: services for deaf and hard of hearing people: issues of equality, participation and access, *Disability and Society*, 16(7): 969–79.

Hearing Concern Link (2008–9) *A Guide to Living with Acquired Profound Hearing Loss*. London: Hearing Concern/Link.

Hogan, A. (2001) *Hearing Rehabilitation for Deafened Adults: A Psychosocial Approach*. London: Whurr.

Lishman, J. (2009) *Communication in Social Work*. Basingstoke: Palgrave.

Morgan-Jones, R.A. (2001) *Hearing Differently: The Impact of Hearing Impairment on Family Life*. London: Whurr.

Moss, B. (2009) *Communication Skills for Health and Social Care*. London: Sage.

Oliver, M. and Sapey, B. (2006) *Social Work with Disabled People*. Basingstoke: Palgrave Macmillan.

Royal National Institute for Deaf People (RNID) (2010) *Your Hearing* http://www.actiononhearingloss.org.uk/your-hearing.aspx, accessed 5 July 2011.

Simmons, M. (2005) *Hearing Loss, from Stigma to Strategy*. London: Peter Owen.

Tait, V. (2007) *Life after Hearing Loss. Telling It Like It Is* . . . London: Hearing Concern.

Trevithick, P. (2005) *Social Work Skills*. Maidenhead: Open University Press.

4   Mental health

Tennyson Mgutshini

Despite the growth of a range of positive mental health initiatives in the last 25 years, injustices and discrimination against those with mental health difficulties remain, and in some areas problems outweigh the progress being made. The exposure to risk of those with mental health difficulties is evident across all areas of everyday life and the stigma associated with the illness limits recovery and adds to the experience of marginalization described by sufferers. This chapter examines the background to this experience of exclusion and increased vulnerability, its nature and concludes by offering potential measures to address this.

Learning objectives

Readers of this chapter will be able to:

- explain how mental health issues represent a domain of risk for adults;
- understand how mental health difficulties can contribute to individual vulnerability in a range of contexts;
- describe the role played by stigma and discrimination in increasing the negative impact that arises from mental health difficulties;
- identify the range and scope of possible interventions to address the marginalization of those with mental health difficulties.

Mental health issues continue to pose practice challenges for both health and social care professionals and the public at large, for related but somewhat different reasons. This is underlined by the wide-ranging and often polarized views and attitudes about how best to respond to this health issue. Much discourse centres on the negative attitudes to mental ill health and divergent views about whether those with mental health difficulties need protection from exploitation by the public or whether the public need to be kept safe from the risks posed by them. Despite this, there is growing acknowledgement that having a mental health difficulty can lead to being marginalized from many day-to-day activities including education, employment and access to public housing. Sayce's (2006) work on exclusion offers a striking illustration of the extent of discrimination faced by those with mental ill health. This recognition of the deeply ingrained disadvantages faced by those with mental health problems represents an important first step in addressing and ameliorating the effects of social exclusion. However, any efforts to address this issue need to be embedded in a clear understanding of the key causative factors behind the exclusion of those with mental ill health.

Mental health: a public and professional challenge

A landmark enquiry by MIND[1] (the National Mental Health Association for England), into the exclusion of those with mental health problems found that most people with mental health problems felt 'excluded from virtually every aspect of society' (MIND 2003). Data for the enquiry was collected by way of a nationwide survey involving 1018 mental health service users, their carers and other stakeholders in mental health, including potential employers and education representatives. In the resulting report, *Creating Accepting Communities*, MIND highlighted specific areas of mainstream life where those with mental health difficulties felt most excluded. With respect to being gainfully employed, an extensive study of employment reported that only 12.9 per cent of people with serious mental health problems were in any form of work (both mainstream and 'sheltered' employment) compared to the national average of 74 per cent found within the general population (Marwaha et al. 2007). From this and other studies, MIND confidently conclude that: 'the entire employment system is underpinned by an unaware but deeply entrenched policy of segregation based on totally false concepts of disability' (2003: 34). The findings from the MIND enquiry suggest high levels of exclusion for those with mental health problems resulting directly from 'labels' attached to their difficulties. The credibility of these assertions lies with the fact that the MIND enquiry, unlike other studies, was based on first-hand reporting by those with mental health difficulties and in that regard offers a rare opportunity for greater awareness of insider perspectives on experiences of exclusion from mainstream society.

Discrimination and stigmatization as causative factors in exclusion

Studies of under-served populations suggest that users of health and social services are vulnerable to exclusion for one or more underlying reasons in addition to their primary vulnerability. These include financial circumstances, place of residence, health, age, functional or developmental status, ability to communicate effectively, race, ethnicity and gender (DoH, 2003; Thornicroft 2006). Most of these characteristics are over-represented among those with mental health problems and as such this group has unique challenges that contribute to their vulnerability to the extent that the social repercussions of having such a condition can be just as harmful as the disease itself (Crisp et al. 2005). Additionally, mental health difficulties have a unique connection with vulnerability in that mental illness can be both a pre-cursor to and a consequence of vulnerability.

At-risk populations often reflect diversity in their social and demographic characteristics such as age, gender, race, ethnicity and socioeconomic status. Considerations of relative vulnerability have historically centred on these characteristics as the primary determinants of individual disadvantage (Honey 2004). Research into the experiences of vulnerable populations (e.g. Walker and Walker 1997; Wilkinson and Marmott 2003; Preston 2005), which adopts a wider approach to understanding vulnerability, asserts that groups of lower socioeconomic status and those from minority ethnic groups experience inherent disadvantages that frequently limit possibilities for equality of access to resources within society. Utilizing either criteria, mental health issues are a source of significant concern to both low socio-economic groups and ethnic minority groups. Contemporary explorations of vulnerability, especially in relation to heterogeneous groups such as those with mental health difficulties urge that attention be turned to meaningful ways of describing vulnerability through understanding the life experiences of the communities and individuals being served, socio-cultural, environmental, economic contexts and community resources, and commonly held attitudes and practices related to a particular group of people.

Reflection on practice

Are individuals with mental health difficulties at risk because they are discriminated *against* or are they at risk because they are victims of discrimination?

Think about your response and consider how this might influence your view about interventions that might reduce vulnerability.

In everyday contexts, the term 'under-served population' is often used inter-changeably with 'vulnerable population'. However, on closer inspection the two terms have some discernable differences. Vulnerability, within the context of health care, is mostly seen as denoting high risk for health and social care problems, while under-served populations are those that specifically receive less health and social care than required for actual or potential health care problems. Even though there is considerable overlap among vulnerable and under-served populations, an individual may be vulnerable and yet not under-served (e.g. a pregnant woman from a minority ethnic group in an intensive care unit and receiving high-quality care). People with mental health problems belong to a rare category of the population that is both under-served *and* vulnerable and at greater risk for adverse health and social outcomes (e.g. financial difficulties, homelessness, suicide, lowered life expectancy; see Table 4.1).

As a result, affected individuals are particularly in need of health and social support.

With specific reference to health, care disparities exist disproportionately in the United Kingdom among under-served populations, the most notable being the homeless (including Gypsies and Travellers – see further Chapter 6), ethnic minorities, people in lower socio-economic groups, with lower educational and reading levels or learning disabilities (see Chapter 5), older people (Chapter 8), and people with physical (Chapter 2) and mental health disabilities (Cooper et al. 2008). Within the context of these broad 'high-vulnerability groups', mental health difficulties are disproportionately over-represented and represent the single common risk area that connects one vulnerable group to the next. In fact, this commonality raises questions about whether one, 'across the board' method of addressing vulnerability would be to increase access to relevant mental health resources and support for all potential and actual service users.

Table 4.1 Health and social indicators of individuals with mental health problems

	People with diagnosed mental health problems	Members of the general population
Life expectancy	63.2 years	79.5 years
Substance and alcohol misuse	30%–60%	10.5%
Risk of being victims of crime	4%	0.5%
Homelessness	12%	0.8%
Unemployment	35%	7.8%

Source: Office of National Statistics, Interim Life Tables, 2009, available at www.statistics.gov.uk/cci.

Discrimination against individuals with mental health difficulties: a public and health conspiracy

There are many negative beliefs about mental health issues found in common discourse today. Public attitudes towards affected individuals range from thinking that they are 'abnormal' to labelling them as 'crazy'. Unlike other health problems, mental health issues tend to be viewed as indicative of a character flaw (the personal deficit model) rather than being compared to other chronic illnesses such as, for example, diabetes. In particular, members of the public (fuelled by the media) tend to associate particular types of mental health difficulties with a range of other moral transgressions such as criminality. The negative impact of these stereotypes, negative attitudes and beliefs is largely uncontested and accounts for many of the exclusions that those with mental health difficulties face. Subjectively, this relationship with society can be particularly detrimental for someone experiencing mental health problems. For example, in the case of someone with depression, associated symptoms of poor self-image and hopelessness are inevitably exacerbated by the negative reactions of those they encounter and further worsen the individual's mental health.

The discrimination encountered by those with mental health is worsened by the fact that it is perpetuated at both organizational and individual level, for example employers are less likely to hire people with known mental health issues. This marginalization is evident in a range of areas within the legal system, for example individuals with diagnosed mental illness have restricted participation on juries, and can be excluded from holding public office by virtue of their illness. The criminal justice system has historically been blamed for unfairly treating those with mental health difficulties in a range of ways including criminalizing mental health by eliciting police rather than mental health professionals' involvement in times of crisis. This has directly impacted on the rates on imprisonment among those with mental health problems.

Insider perspectives on the risks associated with mental health difficulties

Issues relating to the experiences of those with mental health difficulties have historically exclusively been identified within literary sources written by mental health professionals. However, sufferers themselves have offered more recent contributions to the debate about stigma and social exclusion. It is particularly ironic that service users' contributions to the discussion about issues of exclusion and vulnerability have focused primarily on their disenfranchisement within the health care system. Trivedi and Wykes (2002) talk about the prevalence of discrimination they face from mental health professionals by virtue of their diagnosis. Individuals whose views about their illness contradict those of the mental health professional treating them are often labelled as 'lacking insight' into their illness. Insight is seen as a key indicator of treatment success, and those with greatest insight are identified as having a better prognosis than their relatively less insightful peers.

The Sainsbury Centre for Mental Health's (2002) work on treatment concordance, concludes that any patient whose view of their presenting difficulties contradicts that offered by their medical team can in all likelihood expect to be judged as progressively worsening, even if it is reasonable to assume that their personal viewpoint is indeed valuable. This paternalistic view about the ability to self-determine among those with mental health issues further establishes disempowering styles of care which are associated with increased vulnerability and limited personal growth.

Scenario for reflection

Imagine (or, if appropriate, recall) a situation where a health care professional's suggested diagnosis and treatment of a presenting complaint has differed from your own view of what may be occurring.

How would you feel if you expressed alternative views and these were dismissed and attributed to your limited insight into the disorder?

Risk and harm in mental health: a contested issue

The conceptualization of risk within mental health is particularly complex, in part because of the varied perspectives from which this issue has been explored. Mental health problems carry with them associated perceptions of 'difference', perceived as such by both the sufferer and members of the public. The experience of marginalization originates from the point of diagnosis and/or first contact with specialist mental health services. The disempowering impact of being assigned a psychiatric diagnosis is most accurately captured in experiences of war veterans with post-traumatic stress disorder (PTSD). Instead of the expected return back to their countries of origin as heroes, individuals diagnosed with PTSD describe their experiences of marginalization and a loss of social status from war hero to being described as 'weak in the mind'.

Scenario for reflection

Xavier is a 32-year-old veteran who has returned from a two-year deployment in Iraq. He has been newly diagnosed with PTSD and has been attending the local psychiatric acute day treatment service (ADTS) for therapy and to be initiated on mood-stabilizing medication. Since his diagnosis, his general practitioner (GP) has advised Xavier that he is not allowed to drive his car until he has been examined and given clearance by the driving, vehicle and licensing agency (DVLA). Family members have been saying that the war 'scrambled his brain', and instead of feeling like a hero, he sees himself as an outsider. As proof of this, he has even had a local social worker from the Children & Families Team assess him to determine whether he poses a risk to his daughter who lives with him and his wife. To escape this, he has been contemplating applying for redeployment back to Iraq where he is treated like any other soldier. He worries also that he will never get cured like the other patients he meets at the treatment centre who tell him that they have been attending for several years.

(Anonymous excerpt from war veteran log)

Xavier's story is not uncommon as demonstrated by evidence from the United States of America. For many of these returning soldiers the sense of social exclusion associated with their diagnosis may worsen the impact, leading to additional complexities such as substance abuse:

> 'A study of the first 100,000 [Iraq and Afghanistan] veterans seen at Veteran Affairs facilities showed that 25 per cent of them received mental health diagnoses. Of these, 56 per cent had 2 or more mental health diagnoses. The most common were PTSD, substance abuse, and depression'. Evaluation immediately on return from deployment suggested that 5 per cent of active duty and 6 per cent of reserve personnel had a significant mental health problem. When reassessed 3 to 6 months later, 27 per cent of active duty and 42 per cent of reserve personnel received that evaluation.
>
> (USA Public Health Association 2007)

Social integration and mental health diagnosis

The fact that serious mental health problems often have recurrent patterns, by comparison to other illnesses, predisposes affected individuals to have repeated contacts with specialist psychiatric services. In fact, research suggests that between 37 per cent and 53 per cent of people who have contact with psychiatric services require additional specialist intervention within 12 months of their initial contact (Crisp et al. 2005). Unfortunately, service user narratives of contact with specialist psychiatric services provide insights of disempowering and depersonalizing experiences which often leave affected individuals feeling upset, devalued and helpless within a medically dominated system (Mgutshini 2010). By withdrawing the individual from 'normal everyday activity', repeated contact with psychiatric services significantly disrupts integration into community life and, in reality, reduces access to most of the life opportunities available to others such as employment and education. This recurrent contact with psychiatric services is likely to result in the individual service user feeling 'doubly excluded' from normal life, first, as a direct result of the stigma and prejudicial treatment related to being mentally ill, and second, as a result of feeling particularly disadvantaged by 'losing' many of his/her 'productive years' moving in and out of psychiatric facilities.

The latter source of exclusion is blamed for limiting service users' opportunities for real integration into 'normal' existence, to such an extent that the concerned individual's only career prospects may lie in being a 'professional patient' of the psychiatric system (Crowther et al. 2001). In terms of 'social integration' into mainstream community life, individuals with patterns of frequent contact with specialist psychiatric services face an added dimension of exclusion. Most notably, they often only have realistic opportunities for developing relationships with people met within the mental health system at the expense of socially integrating with the wider community within which they will be expected to live.

Mental health problems: debated perceptions of risk

In addition to the generally held view that those with mental health difficulties are themselves vulnerable to discrimination, exclusion and exploitation within public life, an alternate and noteworthy viewpoint is that, on the contrary, the general public need to be protected from those with mental health problems. Within this public protection perspective, often cited within mainstream media, the effects of mental illness are primarily blamed for incidents of violence involving those with mental health difficulties. Much of the basis for this viewpoint emanates from media portrayals of mental ill health – ranging from the Victorian example of the 'insane' who needed detention in asylums to the more recent sensational media depiction of individuals with mental health difficulties.

Further exploration of the alleged danger posed by mentally ill individuals, however, suggest a more complicated picture. In fact, as Graves et al. (2005: 318) indicate:

> The truth is that there is a very strong link between people with mental illnesses and violence – just not the way it generally is portrayed . . . The notion that mentally ill people are dangerous is in fact contrary to the evidence which shows that those with mental health difficulties are actually statistically much more likely to be hurt than to hurt other people.

A 2005 study by researchers at North Western University (USA) confirms this viewpoint in its findings, which showed that up to 25 per cent of people with severe mental illnesses are the victims of violent crime each year. People with mental illness were 23 times more likely to be raped, 15 times more likely to be assaulted, 8 times more likely to be robbed, and were the victims of theft 140 times more often than those in the general population (Teplin and Coon 2005). The findings from this survey are widely accepted as representing the most comprehensive study of victimization ever carried out in relation to mental illness in the world as the sample comprised 32,450 participants. Within the UK, a study published in *The Lancet* concluded that mentally ill patients are six times more likely to be murdered than are people in the general population (Hiroeh et al. 2001). This increased risk of violence, combined with other consequences of exclusion and the impact of illness, all contribute to the picture of substantially high vulnerability among those with mental health difficulties compared to most other health groups.

Regardless of the high rate of victimization experienced by people with mental health problems, serious untoward incidents committed by individuals who may suffer from mental illnesses certainly seize public attention far more that similar incidents committed by members of the general population. Ironically, the fact that reality often reflects an opposite image creates an unexpected blind spot in public perception such that the significant crimes perpetrated against the mentally ill including sexual and financial exploitation receive little or no media coverage.

In addition to the erroneous fears about their danger to society, another common myth is that people with mental illnesses always need to be hospitalized, when in fact they benefit more from care in the community. Although inaccurate, both these beliefs possess significant persuasive power and give impetus to discriminatory attitudes among members of the public. As outsiders, those with mental health problems face an unprecedented range of disadvantages that impact on nearly all aspects of social existence, including employment, housing, within the justice system and in the pursuit of intimate relationships.

Substance misuse: a new dimension in mental health risk

In addition to increased risks of developing a range of physical health problems such as diabetes and coronary heart disease, individuals with mental health problems have a particular vulnerability with respect to substance misuse problems. It is estimated that 30–60 per cent of the psychiatric service user population have an associated problem with substance misuse difficulty compared to estimates of 10–12 per cent within the generic population (Berzins et al. 2003). This increased prevalence of drug- and alcohol-related difficulties is especially relevant as substance misuse represents an added source of vulnerability for varying reasons, including the fact that it further alienates affected individuals from society. 'Excessive substance misuse' is the single most reliable predictor of increased hospitalization risk for people with mental illness, so much so that individuals with additional substance misuse problems present the group with the highest risk of readmission within 30 days after their most recent treatment. Given the increased risks, individuals with substance misuse have an overall poorer prognosis, primarily as a result of being doubly stigmatized by their mental illness and substance use problems.

Stigma and marginalization: wide-ranging effects on vulnerability

The stigma of mental health difficulties acts as an important deterrent to acknowledging need for specialist psychiatric interventions. This has been especially reported with respect to war veterans who are likely to under-report the severity of their post-traumatic stress symptoms to avoid the stigma that comes with admitting a psychiatric illness. Similarly, the reluctance to seek out treatment by those with mental health difficulties has been attributed to this fear of being stigmatized. Such is the severity of this fear of stigma that many choose to suffer through the anguish of a mental illness rather than risk being labelled as 'mentally ill'. Evidence of this is most notable with respect to employment issues despite the fact that anti-discriminatory legislation such as the Disability Discrimination Act (2005) and (Single) Equalities Act (2010) in the UK; and the Americans with Disabilities Act (1990), make provision for a range of accommodations to be made to protect those with mental health difficulties in the areas of employment, education and housing. The legislative changes have largely failed to establish themselves as a strong enough reassurance for sufferers that they will be protected from the harmful effects of stigma and discrimination. Access to employment is a significant protection against poverty, homelessness and a range of other exclusions. Accordingly, practical interventions are required to destigmatize mental health issues within employment and to support existing legislation and policies.

Addressing issues of risk relating to mental health

Combating exclusion and discrimination: a priority for mental health

In the UK, the strategy for combating discriminatory attitudes towards mental health issues focuses on a number of areas, including increasing public awareness and understanding of the need for positive mental health and well-being. In Britain the government produced a *National Service Framework for Mental Health* (DoH 1999), which focuses on the mental health needs of adults of working age, up to the age of 65. The Framework has a number of guiding values and principles, including the involvement of service users and their carers in the planning and delivery of care, the promotion of joint working between agencies that deliver care, including health and social care services as well as the voluntary sector, and ensuring that service users are supported with integration issues.

It is clear that many of the risks of harm faced by those with mental health problems are largely a consequence of the stigma, social exclusion and discrimination they experience in every aspect of their social and personal life. Other contributory factors include the fact that provision for mental health issues continues to be largely reactive and insufficient to proactively address the growing population of people with mental health difficulties in the United Kingdom. Any action to address the vulnerabilities of those mental health difficulties should focus on positive mental health initiatives and measures to eliminate the stigma of mental illness. Furthermore, a need exists for mental health services that empower rather than dis-empower service users. The foundation for such work should be based on the acknowledgement that a failure to eliminate stigma and discrimination of those with mental health problems would impact on 25 per cent of mainstream population given that one in four people experience mental health difficulties during at least one point in their lifetime.

Traditional approaches to addressing stigmatization and social exclusion have focused primarily on interventions intended to redefine public or community perceptions about mental illness (Thornicroft 2006). By contrast, limited attention has been given to challenging organizational barriers that individuals have to overcome, with regard to accessing justice, accommodation, employment and even with engaging with professionals providing care to them within the mental health system. Given the role of mental health professionals in advocating for more inclusive attitudes towards mental health, the initial recognition of the sources of discrimination for those with psychiatric illnesses should be a primary priority for any efforts that address discrimination. To assist professionals (both working in mental health and in a range of other agencies) in this advocacy role, the Engagement Matrix (Figure 4.1) identifies the key areas of vulnerability and risk to which those with mental health difficulties are exposed.

For professionals seeking to address disadvantage and risk, it is important to ensure that a comprehensive implementation of interventions ensues to minimize the negative impact on individuals with mental health needs. For example, clinicians should ensure that involuntary hospitalization occurs only when absolutely necessary and that, when hospitalized, individuals do not become isolated or depersonalized. In particular, they should receive treatment that encourages individual expression. At practice level, this implies countering the discrimination that often affects people once they start to use mental health services. Ramon's (1991: 6) work with individuals with learning difficulties advocates for 'normalization or social role valorization', a principle in which practitioners recognize that patients have the right to 'lead a valued ordinary life, based on the belief in equality as human beings and citizens'. This theoretical framework aims to produce a situation where people with mental health difficulties occupy valued social roles and experience themselves as valuable, competent people whose health care choices will be appreciated and not dismissed by virtue of the assumed diminished competence often attributed to their illness.

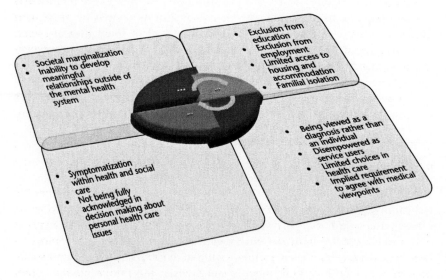

Figure 4.1 The Engagement Matrix.

Source: © Mgutshini (2010).

Scenarios for reflection

The literature suggests that, as individuals, both clinicians and members of the public hold discriminatory attitudes towards mental health issues. Think about your own beliefs and identify two myths about mental health that you are aware of. Is there reliable evidence to support these beliefs?

If you are a current practitioner, identify areas of discrimination for people with mental health difficulties in the professional area in which you work (use the Engagement Matrix as a guide).

Select three priority areas and devise a plan (or set of strategies) to address each of your identified challenges.

Challenging social attitudes: the public agenda

Challenges that arise from discrimination and social exclusion are not confined to people who have experienced mental health distress but also impact on their families, carers, friends and significant others. As a result, action to address the stigma of mental illness not only benefits those who suffer from the condition, but can help to ensure that the communities in which they live will prosper, as greater numbers of citizens experience more productive relationships and are able to support the affected individual to live as independently as possible.

Dating back as far as 1991, there has been a global acceptance that there is a need to combat the stigma and discrimination experienced by those with mental health problems. The United Nation General Assembly's policy paper, 'Principles for the protection of persons with mental illness and the improvement of mental health care' (United Nations 1991) identifies four specific areas where focus should be placed in addressing issues of stigma, social exclusion and the re-integration of those with mental health problems. Table 4.2 provides an overview of possible actions to address discrimination and marginalization.

Challenging misconceptions and inaccurate portrayals of mental health issues

The stigma and discrimination within different sectors of society are often the result of misconception and myths about mental illness. In turn these are expressed as discriminatory attitudes and behaviour. Attitudes and portrayals of those suffering from mental illness, in particular schizophrenia, depict it as an illness, which increases the tendency for violence. People from lower socio-economic groups including mentally ill Gypsies and Travellers and other ethnic minorities are especially vulnerable to discrimination as members of already marginalized social groups (O'Hara 2010).

Table 4.2 Actions for engaging with discrimination and marginalization

1. Challenging misconceptions about mental health issues	• Educational initiatives with adolescents, law enforcement, health and social care providers. • Advocating for media images that promote more accurate perceptions of mental health issues. • Facilitating events that facilitate direct interaction between sufferers and members of the public.
2. Effective treatments	• Developing initiatives to educate those with mental health problems about the range of treatments and support interventions available to them. • Advocating for mental health promotion with at-risk populations and members of the general public.
3. Employment and support	• Developing relationships with industry and employers to educate them about mental health issues and to negotiate employment partnerships. • Exploring and facilitating the development of wider options for meaningful daytime occupation. • Advocating for further action to support the anti-discriminatory measures within the Disability Discrimination Act (2005).
4. The development of positive media drives	• Advocating for responsible media portrayals of mental health. • Negotiating media partnerships with mass media to publish educational content about mental health issues.

Examples of common myths:

• Mental health problems increase an individual's tendency towards violent and aggressive behaviour.
• Mental health difficulties are a result of a character flaw and cannot be treated.

Addressing misconceptions through education and other attitude modification approaches is one of the most important ways of tackling prejudice and discriminatory views. In particular, media sources can lead in this regard – the media, through portraying mental health issues accurately, and the government, through developing initiatives, increase awareness and normalize the experience mental illness.

Examples of interventions which challenge negative attitudes towards
mental health issues

Example 1

Changing Minds – Every Family in the Land (Royal College of Psychiatrists 2002)

Initially developed in 1998, this was a five-year rolling programme developed jointly by the Royal College of Psychiatrists and the Office of National Statistics to change public opinion concerning six types of mental illness (anxiety disorders, depression, schizophrenia, dementia, eating disorders and substance misuse). It addressed negative attitudes found among particular groups such as medical practitioners, children and adolescents and the general (adult) population. The primary focus of the initiative was to improve understanding and communication between sufferers, clinicians and health care workers utilizing a range of media including film, video and open discussion.

An assessment of public participant attitudes pre- and post-engagement with the initiative revealed an improvement in attitudes towards people suffering from the listed conditions.

Example 2

Open the Doors

'Open the Doors' is an international programme initiated in 1996 by the World Psychiatric Association. It focuses on combating negative attitudes about schizophrenia. Over 14 years later, it now exists in over 25 countries in Africa, Europe, North and South America and has resulted in 200 anti-stigma interventions with a priority of awareness building and attitude modification. The programme has four distinct features that separate it from other initiatives:

1. Focus on schizophrenia.
2. Close collaboration between mental health services, service users, families and clinicians.
3. Interventions are specifically targeted towards journalists, law enforcement, general practitioners, secondary school students and government officials.
4. The global nature of the programme offers advantages in that varied approaches have been developed to work with diverse populations (WHO 2002; Stuart 2008).

Employment and support

One of the key areas where inclusion of those with mental health difficulties should be promoted is within employment. Research suggests that work of some kind has both preventative and rehabilitative effects for people with mental health problems and represents an important measure of full citizenship and normality (Marwaha et al. 2007). It is important too to stress that employment in this context refers to both paid and unpaid activities as for some people with mental health difficulties, unpaid alternatives such as volunteering, training and other satisfying activities may be more fulfilling and realistically sustainable than paid work where a range of expectations or responsibilities may exist which may impact negatively on the individual in times of illness.

Despite broad agreement about the benefits of some kind of employment, barriers to such activities exist for people with mental health difficulties. Broadly speaking, these fall into three categories:

- *Internalized barriers*: including low self-confidence, and feelings of being deskilled;
- *Structural*: organizational restrictions and the state of the employment market;
- *Attitudinal*: negative beliefs (of others) that limit the potential for people with mental health difficulties.

The creation of employment opportunities that could suitably engage people who may be vulnerable in stressful work environments is an issue which governments, corporate entities and society as a whole need to address as a social justice responsibility.

As a starting point, mental health professionals, with the support of the government and existing legislation (e.g. the Disability Act 1995 and the Equality Act 2010) should participate in activities that challenge employers to develop positive attitudes towards mental health issues within the workplace. Advocacy by mental health professionals can take a variety of forms, ranging from educating the public, demystifying mental health issues and protesting against inaccurate media portrayals.

Chapter summary

- Mental health issues are largely misunderstood and, as a result, affected individuals and their families face stigmatization, exclusion and discrimination in a wide range of areas in everyday life.

- The discrimination and social exclusion faced by those with mental health issues is a source of disadvantage and increases vulnerability to poorer health, increased risk of violence from the public, isolation and worse prognosis in most health and social care categories.

- As a result of increased vulnerability, those with mental health difficulties live comparatively shorter lives than members of the general public, have increased risk of substance misuse, have increased rates of homelessness and unemployment and are discriminated against within the criminal justice system.

- Discrimination continues even within the health care system, where those with mental health difficulties feel disempowered as service users.

- 'Normalization' is an important principle, which recognizes that individuals with mental health difficulties have a right to lead a valued 'ordinary' life based on equality as human beings and citizens.

Note

1   MIND is the leading Mental Health Association that represents service users and their carers in England and is acknowledged by user groups, policy makers and service providers as the primary voice for service users.

References

Berzins, K., Petch, A. and Atkinson, J. (2003) Prevalence and experience of harassment of people with mental health problems living in the community. *The British Journal of Psychiatry*, 826–33.

Cooper, C., Morgan, C., Byrne, M., Dazzan, P. et al. (2008) Perceptions of disadvantage, ethnicity, and psychosis. *The British Journal of Psychiatry*, 192: 185–90.

Crisp, A., Gedder, M., Goddard, E. et al. (2005) Stigmatization of people with mental illness: a follow-up study within the 'Changing Minds' campaign of the Royal College of Psychiatrists. *World Psychiatry*, 4: 106–13.

Crowther, R.E., Marshall, M., Bond, G.R. et al. (2001) Helping people with severe mental illness to obtain work: systematic review. *British Medical Journal*, 3221: 204–8.

Department of Health (DoH) (1999) *National Service Framework for Mental Health*. London: DoH.

Department of Health (DoH) (2003) *Attitudes to Mental Illness*. London: DoH.

Graves, R., Cassisi, J. and Penn, D. (2005) Psycho-physiological evaluation of stigma towards schizophrenia. *Schizophrenia Research*, 76: 317–27.

Hiroeh, U., Appleby, L., Mortensen, P. and Dunn, G. (2001) Death by homicide, suicide and other unnatural causes in people with mental illness: a population based study: *The Lancet*, 358(9299): 2110–14.

Honey, A. (2004) Benefits and drawbacks of employment: perspectives of people with mental illness. *Qualitative Research*, 14: 381–95.

Marwaha, S., Johnson, S., Bebbington, P. et al. (2007) Rates and correlates of employment in people with schizophrenia in the UK, France and Germany. *The British Journal of Psychiatry*, 191: 30–7.

Mgutshini, T. (2010) Risk factors for psychiatric re-hospitalization (an exploration). *International Journal of Mental Health Nursing*, 19: 321–36.

MIND (2003) *The Report on the MIND Report: 'Creating Accepting Communities'*. London: MIND.

O'Hara, M. (2010) (News report) Fightback over claims on mental illness and its prevalence among black people. *Guardian*, 3 February.

Preston, G. (ed.) (2005) *At Greatest Risk: The Children Most Likely to Be Poor*. London: Child Poverty Action Group.

Ramon, S. (1991) *Beyond Community Care: Normalisation and Integration Work*. London: Macmillan.

Royal College of Psychiatrists (RCP) (2002) *Changing Minds: Our Lives and Mental Illness*. London: RCP Publishing.

Sainsbury Centre for Mental Health (2002) *Breaking the Circles of Fear: A Review of the Relationship between Mental Health Services and African and Caribbean Communities*. London: Sainsbury Centre for Mental Health.

Sayce, L. (2006) *From Psychiatric Patient to Citizen: Overcoming Discrimination and Social Exclusion*. London: Palgrave.

Seeker, J., Grove, B. and Seebohm, P. (2001) Challenging barriers to employment, training and education for mental health service users: the service user's perspective. *Journal of Mental Health*, 10: 395–404.

Stuart, H. (2008) Fighting the stigma caused by mental disorders: past perspectives, present activities, and future directions. *World Psychiatry*, 7(3): 185–88.

Teplin, L. and Coon, O. (2005) *The National Victimization Survey (NCVS), Bureau of Justice Statistics*. Chicago, IL: Bureau of Justice.

Thornicroft, G. (2006) *Shunned: Discrimination Against People with Mental Illness*. Oxford: Oxford University Press.

Thornicroft, G., Rose, D., Kassam, K. and Sartorius, N. (2007) Stigma, ignorance, prejudice or discrimination. *The British Journal of Psychiatry*, 190: 192–4.

Trivedi, P. and Wykes, T. (2002) From passive subjects to equal partners: qualitative review of user involvement in research. *The British Journal of Psychiatry*, 181: 468–72.

United Nations (1991) *Principles for the Protection of Persons with Mental Illness and the Improvement of Mental Health Care*. Geneva: Office of the United Nations High Commissioner for Human Rights.

USA Public Health Association (2007) 135th annual meeting: abstract 165759, 5 November.

Walker, A. and Walker, C. (eds) (1997) *Britain Divided: The Growth of Social Exclusion in the 1980s and 1990s*. London: CPAG.

Wilkinson, R. and Marmott, M. (2003) *The Social determinants of Health: The Solid Facts*, Geneva: The International Centre for Health and Society.

World Health Organization (2002) *Close the Gap: Dare to Care*. Geneva: World Health Organization.

5   Learning disability

Michael Farquharson and Jill Aitken

People with a learning disability (LD) are commonly recognized as being at risk of harm. Epilepsy is a condition that many individuals have to contend with in addition to their learning disability. Generally, practitioners recognize that in order to support people with LD and ensure that innate vulnerabilities do not expose them to further risk or actual harm (e.g., homelessness, abuse as an older person and exploitation), a coherent, responsive and individualized package of support is required. This chapter aims to explore the ways in which legislation and policy recommendations can be used to ensure that people with a LD are empowered and supported in life choices. These life choices must be in the individual's best interests and yet recognize their dignity and capacity to participate in their own care decisions wherever possible.[1]

Two case scenarios will be referred to throughout the chapter to illustrate the concepts introduced. These case studies are those of individuals whose LD obliges them to access a range of services including health and social care provision in a community setting. The chapter highlights the challenges for practitioners in promoting the well-being for individuals with LD which includes ensuring that those requiring support do not suffer exclusion from mainstream services and therefore an increased vulnerability, at any stage in their lifespan.

Learning objectives

Readers of this chapter will be able to:

- comprehend the specific vulnerabilities experienced by people with hidden disabilities;
- understand the ways in which having a learning disability (LD) is related to epilepsy; the risks associated with each and the exacerbated vulnerabilities which arise when concurrent impairments are found;

- enhance awareness of the risks of stigmatization and the ways in which exclusion may occur for people with LD and epilepsy;
- develop a heightened awareness of the way in which legislative and policy enactments are able to empower individuals when practitioners are engaged with people with LD and epilepsy.

Learning disability: definitions and incidence

The potential vulnerability of individuals with LD is frequently attested, most recently in Department of Health (2001, 2004) circulars and in a MENCAP (2007) report. The effects of LD on the individual and their family are extensive and the vulnerabilities that arise from this condition are broader than might at first be thought. There are various definitions of LD, but perhaps the most commonly used are those arrived at in policy documents and Department of Health reports of the last decade. The first such definition of LD is a legal one, provided by the Mental Health Bill (2006) which refers to this group of people, using different terminology, as having a mental retardation. The Mental Health Bill (2006) notes that 'mental retardation is a condition of arrested or incomplete development of the mind characterized by impairment of skills and overall intelligence in areas such as cognition, language, and motor and social abilities'. The second definition originates from *Valuing People* (DoH 2001) which affords more detail and identifies three separate human characteristic points arguing that a 'learning disability includes the presence of:

- A significantly reduced ability to understand new or complex information, to learn new skills (impaired intelligence), with;
- A reduced ability to cope independently (impaired social functioning);
- Which started before adulthood, has a lasting effect on development'.

The spectrum of cognitive impairments covered by the general term LD is a broad and nuanced one and Alborz et al. (2005) argue that the physical, as well as the cognitive abilities of a person with a LD may differ greatly. The difference in level of needs comes via the level of support necessary to be a participant in successful daily living.

The exact prevalence of people with a LD in the United Kingdom is difficult to gauge as there is a lack of comprehensive data available. The reported incidence of LD within the total population also varies from one source of data to another. However, some of the most commonly quoted estimates is contained in *Valuing People* (DoH 2001) which suggests that there were approximately 1.4 million people with LD in England at the turn of the 21st century. Of this group 1.2 million had mild LD and 210,000 had a severe or profound LD. The number of people within the UK as a whole is generally rounded up to 1.5 million. As with all estimates there are discrepancies; however, these statistics demonstrate the range of LD and therefore the possible prevalence of associated health concerns (that often include epilepsy).

More recently, Emerson and Hatton (2004) estimated that the current and future number of people with a LD in England was 985,000; 2 per cent of the general population. The difference in estimations between Emerson and Hatton and DoH (2001) results from the higher mortality rate in LD, where life expectancy is reduced in comparison with others. Emerson and Hatton (2008) further suggest that this is evident in a reduced ratio of the older portion of people with LD. NICE (2010–11) notes that people with a LD are 58 times more likely to die before the age of 50 than the general population.

The future prevalence of LD challenges service providers. Predicted demographic changes for the general population of England will inescapably lead to an increase in the number of adults with a LD. However, other factors will also contribute to an increase, including improved survival rates of young people with severe and complex disabilities, reduced mortality of older adults with LD and the increased proportion of younger English adults emanating from South Asian ethnic minority communities, where prevalence rates are higher (NICE 2010–11). Michaels and Richardson (2008) also predict the incidence of LD rising by 1 per cent per year for the next 10 years and that there will also be a growth in the complexity of disabilities. MENCAP (2004) purports that in addition there is likely to be a higher prevalence of some additional medical conditions or concerns, with epilepsy being one of those.[2]

Legislative safeguards for those with LD

Policy initiatives to address social exclusion and vulnerability have progressed in recent years, yielding important legislation to protect and empower those with LD. One of these is the Mental Capacity Act (2005) which enables those with LD to become more active arbiters of their own lives.[3] However, the Mental Capacity Act also highlights and describes other individuals or groups of vulnerable adults such as those who have a physical or sensory disability, including those people who are physically frail or have a chronic illness; those who have a mental illness, including dementia; those who have a LD; those who are old; those who are dependent upon drugs or alcohol; and those who have social or emotional problems, or whose behaviour challenges services. The Mental Capacity Act also identifies 'people with grave physical conditions, who may experience confusion, drowsiness or loss of consciousness as a result of their illness or treatment'.

For many years those providing services to people with LD have held the responsibility of promoting issues that surround this client group, in other words, choices, equality and their diverse needs. How the Mental Capacity Act (2005) is interpreted and utilized is essential when providing packages of care for people with a LD. The aim of LD practitioners and service providers is to provide high-quality health and social care services for people with a LD which enables and supports the individual to participate in the activities of everyday life. This participation empowers the individual, providing choices and opportunities that give them similar chances and options to their non-LD counterparts. The addition of a dual diagnosis (often epilepsy) or other conditions makes this process more complex; however, any additional problem can be ameliorated to a great extent by best professional practice.

A person's vulnerability will depend on their circumstances and environment, and each case must be judged on its own merits. Is it right to assume that all those who have a LD are vulnerable or does such an assumption risk making choices for such people without truly recognizing individual self-determination? The Human Rights Act (1998) states that all individuals have the right to live free from the fear of harm. This is where the Mental Capacity Act (2005) provides structure and insight into individual need and provides a code of practice to define the subjects that this Act seeks to protect. Similarly, if the following principles are applied, a person must be assumed to have capacity unless it is established that they lack capacity; that the person is not to be treated as unable to make a decision unless all practicable steps to assist them to do so have been taken without success. Further to this, a person is not to be considered as unable to make a decision merely because they might make an unwise decision. The Mental Capacity Act also stipulates that acts done or decisions made for, or on behalf of a person who lacks capacity must be done, or made, in their best interests. Before the act is done, or the decision made, there must be thought as to whether the purpose for which it is needed can be as effectively achieved in a manner less restrictive of the individual's rights and freedom of action.

Clearly the Mental Capacity Act (2005) does not apply solely to the field of LD but instead ranges across the spectrum of recognized impairments and disabilities. However, Wong et al. (2000) highlight the increased volume of incapacity in adults with a LD, as compared to the general population therefore indicating the centrality of the Mental Capacity Act (2005) in the care of this particular group of people. Similarly, Keywood et al. (1999) warn of the innate readiness to assume that those with a LD lack the ability to contribute to the decision-making process. However, the Mental Capacity Act addresses these issues to a certain extent by encouraging the identification of capacity and how this legislation should be implemented within practice. This guidance indicates how practitioners can be self-regulating in practice by questioning any decisions made and the manner that conclusions are formulated. Those with a LD are also protected by the same legislation as other groups within the UK.

In order to demonstrate the psychosocial impact of a LD on the health of an individual the use of case studies will be employed. Case studies consist of 'real life' situations but service users' names have to be changed to preserve confidentiality.

Scenario for reflection 1

Richard is a 57-year-old man who lives at home with his elderly mother (aged 90). He is the youngest of three children and is autistic. Richard attended mainstream school until the age of 11 when he was transferred to a school in a LD institution to finish his education. He then attended a Day Centre for a short while but then dropped out of 'services' when this facility closed and has not received any support for many years. Richard is morbidly obese and has leg ulcers and respiratory problems. He cannot wash himself adequately and his mother is now unable to help him. Richard rarely goes out at all mainly because of his obesity and leg ulcers so has difficulty in walking any distance. He doesn't like crowds or what he considers a lot of noise. He rarely maintains eye contact or holds any discussion but does converse quite well when he is in the mood to do so. This is usually pretty brief as he spends a lot of his time in his bedroom avoiding too much contact with anybody. Richard does not have any friends, however, he does have imaginary friends that he talks to quite regularly. Richard is rather concrete-thinking and takes things literally. He lacks imagination and does not recognize or really consider other people's feelings, neither is he able to express his own. Richard gives the impression that he understands situations and details when he doesn't. He does not like to admit that he doesn't 'understand' as he feels that it is easier to say 'yes' rather than 'no' when asked. He finally came to the attention of the LD services as an outcome of a hospital admission for his respiratory problems, the concerns of his older siblings and as a result of police reports in the wake of harassment by local youths, who threw missiles at his bedroom window.

The importance of personalization

The Mental Capacity Act (2005) requires that in Scenario 1 the health and social care practitioners, respect, actively include and listen to Richard in the decision-making process while at the same time taking account of the need to safeguard their own professional practice. Within LD it is important to view the whole individual, and priority must be given to recognizing the everyday challenges confronting and surrounding the person and assist them in negotiating these in a structured and supported manner. In so doing practice must be meticulous and person-centred. Planning for the care of individuals should include a delicate balance of risk assessment, personalized care, and fastidious cost-benefit analysis. At different levels of LD, it may be necessary for more support: those with profound LD may be more reliant on support agents than others and are often known to statutory services and receive a high level of support. It is also well reported that those who go unnoticed by local and statutory services are often those whose LD are mild and who are functioning 'well' without support or with total support by family members or significant others, a situation evident in Scenario 1.

Richard can certainly be considered to be a vulnerable adult with a LD but for many years had not been 'noticed' by the appropriate services. This was probably due to a state of denial on behalf of his mother who considered him to be 'a little backward'. As Richard was 'unknown' to the local LD services he required a full needs assessment to be completed. This assessment necessitates a multi-disciplinary approach involving a psychologist, care manager, dietician, general practitioner and psychiatrist, practice nurses, social worker, police and direct care staff. Perhaps more importantly, Richard, his mother and siblings needed to be central to the whole process. In this scenario it is not simply the treatment that impacts on the individual, but the support networks and degree of understanding of those health and social care professionals dedicated to their care. In this respect, the NICE (2004) guidelines provide best evidence and best practice recommendations, acknowledging that people matter – in this scenario Richard and his mother – more than systems and that person-centred planning 'starts' from the person's perspective. Best practice must include working with the person's circle of support and must be driven by the totality of the person's life, allowing them to achieve the best possible quality of life.

Vulnerability of living with a learning disability

In Scenario 1 Richard was fully involved in the planning of his care. Great consideration was taken to explain plans in terms that Richard would understand, in accordance with the requirements of the Mental Capacity Act (2005). Initially it was decided that his safety and immediate physical needs should be met as a priority. A two-pronged approach was planned: first, the community Police Officer in accordance with their *Safeguarding Vulnerable Adults* strategy organized the instalment of specialist 'safety' and deterrent (additional locks, lights and alarms) equipment to the house to ensure that both Richard and his mother felt more secure. Police authorities have well-published guidelines for the management of such circumstances. Highlighting the vulnerability of people with LD, research entitled *Living in Fear* (MENCAP 2000) found that nearly 9 out of 10 people with LD had been either harassed or attacked within the last year, with 32 per cent reported that they experienced harassment or attacks on a daily or weekly basis. Twenty-three per cent had actually been assaulted at some point (Figure 5.1). There have also been several well-reported cases of murder purely because the victim had a LD. Police guidelines now provide mandatory training for all frontline officers in procedures to reduce and manage such crimes, even those that might appear inconsequential because a series of minor disability hate crimes may dramatically escalate.

In similar vein, *Getting Away with Murder* (Scope 2008) highlights some of the worst case scenarios of hate crime against people with disabilities. It provides real insight into the level of risk that people with LD are facing and confirms the need for acknowledgement of LD as a vulnerable adult.

The vulnerability of people with a LD can also be evident in accessing and receiving appropriate physical and social health care. People with LD often experience poorer health and are twice as likely to be admitted to hospital. Their health needs can go unrecognized, which has an impact on both quality of life and life expectancy (NICE 2010–11). Health remains one of the three priorities for the government's LD strategy. Therefore the second and concur-rent action included greater attention to Richard's medical requirements, respi-ratory problems and leg ulcers, help with personal hygiene, mobility assistance within the home in the form of hand rails on the stairs etc. and, importantly,

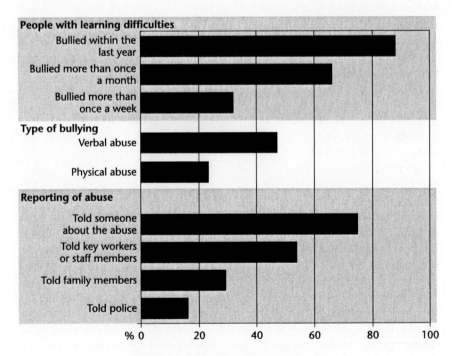

Figure 5.1   Disability hate crime in the UK.
Source: MENCAP (2000)

specialist dietetic intervention. These physical requirements had predominantly gone unnoticed to date and little specialist intervention had been
received until his admission for acute respiratory problems. However, the
Equality Act (2010) gives disabled people rights not to be discriminated against
in access to health services and social services. Importantly, in Scenario 1 this
also includes the services provided at doctors' surgeries and hospitals. While
Richard had received good care during his hospital admission, his ongoing
management by the local surgery had been rather meagre. His hospital care had
been enhanced by the LD liaison nurse who had ensured that Richard had
received appropriate care by checking that reasonable adjustments were in
place throughout his stay. The Equality Act (2010) states that adjustments have
to be made to enable accessing of services, where it is reasonable for the service
provider to make these adjustments. This might include the provision of information about health care in a format that is accessible to the person with a LD.

Empowerment to reduce vulnerability

As noted earlier, it is important to heed the voice of people with LD. To achieve
this, consideration must be paid to the choices, wishes, needs and desires of
learning disabled people (and their families) in their everyday lives. This recognition of the centrality of the individual promotes respect and protection of
the rights, interests and entitlements of people with LD, and it is through this
process of empowerment that dignity and quality of life can be optimized and
vulnerability reduced. Therefore the notion of empowerment, although rather
nebulous, is fundamental to provision of care in LD. However, Dempsey and
Foreman (1997) suggest that there are both explicit and implicit similarities
between various different definitions and that these can be formalized into
seven core components of empowerment:

- self-efficacy: the individual's belief that a situation may be changed or
  influenced;
- participation and collaboration: a collaborative relationship between
  the person that needs help and those giving it;
- sense of control: change is attributed to the actions of the person
  concerned;
- meeting personal needs: the needs and aspirations of the person are
  addressed in a manner which promotes capability and competence;
- understanding the environment: the person is capable of making a
  critical analysis of the services, structures and sources of (both formal
  and informal) support in their environment;
- personal action: there are opportunities to express empowerment in
  diverse ways;

- access to resources: including acute and community services, friends and relatives, community groups and organizations as appropriate.

To empower Richard the Care Manager made arrangements for additional financial benefits to be claimed to facilitate assistance with his hygiene requirements. Richard and his mother were visited by three separate care providers and were able to choose the most appropriate: having made this choice, arrangements were made for a carer to call each day. Both Richard and his mother were happy with the opportunity to exert some choice and control of their circumstances. The situation was ongoing at the time of writing but all concerned are working with Richard and together as a team to secure the best possible outcomes.

(NB. Future plans include greater socialization as agreed with Richard and plans for care when his mother is unable to support his every day needs or on her demise.)

Scenario for reflection 2

Stephen is 32 years old and was born with a LD. He was actively encouraged to involve himself as much as possible with all activities of daily living. As a young man Stephen had 'mild' LD and was coping well but as a result of a road traffic accident he developed epilepsy. The changes were catastrophic. Overnight Stephen's independence 'disappeared' and he was not able to participate in activities that had previously been a natural part of his everyday life. The change was difficult for Stephen to manage and there were changes not only to his lifestyle, but to his behaviour also. The onset of epilepsy meant a variety of things for both the onlooker and individual. In his new role as a person with epilepsy, Stephen was vulnerable and this was evident in particular behaviours. Stephen began to use his epilepsy as a means of control and could have seizures in any given situation that provided a means of controlling that situation. It was not unknown for him to have seizures in the middle of the road, when new members of the multi-disciplinary team were allocated to support him or when a decision was made to change some activity within his life. However, on occasions when the activity or the consequence involved what he considered as important, then seizure frequency could be dramatically reduced. Now at 32 he is in the process of moving into independent living accommodation and there has been a sudden increase in seizure frequency. This has created changes to quality of life as a result of his epilepsy. This example highlights a group of issues around stigma for the practitioner and demonstrates the working impact and knowledge necessary to support and enable this young man.

Epilepsy: definitions and incidence

Stephen has epilepsy, which is commonly found in LD. Epilepsy is the most common, serious, neurological condition and is defined as a tendency to experience recurrent seizures and can affect anyone at any age (Joint Epilepsy Council 2005). Seizures are produced by a sudden burst of excess electrical activity in the brain, which by its nature will often mean that there is no warning of the seizure. There are approximately 40 different types of seizure and a person may have more than one type (Joint Epilepsy Council 2005). The suddenness of epilepsy will therefore place the individual in a more vulnerable position than those who have other long-term conditions (DoH 2004). This greater vulnerability can be created in several ways. Kerr and Wilcox (2006) found that people with epilepsy and LD have a greater risk of accidents and hospitalization, while the rate of limb fractures was double that of those who only had a LD. Perhaps more alarmingly, the risk of death as a result of epilepsy should be highlighted. SUDEP (Sudden Unexplained [or unexpected] Death in Epilepsy) is the most prevalent cause of seizure-related deaths in patients with epilepsy (Morton et al. 2006). The widely accepted definition of SUDEP is 'sudden, unexpected, witnessed or unwitnessed, nontraumatic and nondrowning death in patients with epilepsy, with or without evidence for a seizure, and excluding documented status epilepticus, in which post-mortem examination does not reveal a toxicological or anatomic cause for death' (Nashef 1997). A series of factors were identified as contributing to increase risk. Some of these include polypharmacy, dose change and compliance, all of which can be found within LD (Beran et al. 2004; Hitiris et al. 2007). Risk is further exacerbated by recent diagnosis, intractable epilepsy, nocturnal and tonic clonic seizures (Tompson et al. 2005). Once these facts are recognized, it can be concluded that an increased level of risk is possible for persons with LD and epilepsy.

Approximately 50 million people worldwide are affected with epilepsy (International League Against Epilepsy/International Bureau for Epilepsy/World Health Organization 2003) and 1 in 131 people in the United Kingdom (Epilepsy Action 2009). It is estimated that about 460,000 people in England and Wales, in other words, 1 per cent of the population, have epilepsy in one form or another. This figure demonstrates the real impact of epilepsy within the UK.

Concomitance of learning disability and epilepsy

The incidence of epilepsy is higher in the population of people with LD. This link, or association, is generally accepted to be as a result of the underlying brain disorder or damage that is evident in both LD and epilepsy (Espie et al. 2003; Matthews et al. 2008). The actual incidence is difficult to pinpoint however. Kerr et al. (2009) estimate that the number is in the region of 32 per cent of those with LD while Lhatoo and Sander (2001) argue 1 in 5. Nonetheless, most sources agree that the prevalence of people with epilepsy and LD increases the more severe the LD and this can be as much as 1 in 2 people with profound and multiple LD (DoH 2001). These statistics present striking data and demonstrate the importance of a full understanding of epilepsy and its effects within the LD population.

Learning point

One to two per cent of the population have some degree of LD. This translates to up to 30 per cent of people with LD having epilepsy, rising to up to 50 per cent for those with a severe LD. This demonstrates the impact and co-morbidity issues that surround this dual diagnosis.

Reuber (2007, cited in All Party Parliamentary Group on Epilepsy (APPG) 2007) suggests that the mean proportion of people with epilepsy and LD who achieved seizure-control was between 22 and 32.8 per cent – significantly below the proportion of the general population with epilepsy. The APPG recommendation was that the Department of Health and the Department for Education and Skills, should take steps to deliver the NICE guidance on the treatment of people with epilepsy with LD and issue a guidance note to epilepsy health professionals on how to meet the NICE guidance. Beavis et al. (2007) and Loughran and O'Brien (2001) have found that it is difficult to attain seizure freedom in those with LD, as far too often their epilepsy is complex and this group are more predisposed to having refractory epilepsy than any other group within epilepsy. When compiling care and treatment plans, this limited ability to achieve seizure freedom means that monotherapy is often not achievable and so it is common to see polytherapy (the use of three or more drugs) (Kerr et al. 2009). Lanfear (2002) believes that the aim of any treatment is control of seizures without unacceptable side effects that promote good quality of life and psychological well-being.

Quality of life

The term 'quality of life' is used to evaluate the general well-being of individuals and societies. It is used in a wide range of contexts, including the fields of health care. The standard indicators of the quality of life include environmental elements, physical and mental health, recreation and leisure time, and social belonging. The link between social value and social exclusion can be seen in the International League Against Epilepsy (ILAE) definition of quality of life: 'an individual's emotional response to their life circumstances, the gap between these circumstances and their expectations and their ability to meet their personal needs' (ILAE/IBE/WHO 2003: 57). Leplege and Hunt (1997) describe issues that create concerns within quality of life, as linking to people's emotional, social and physical well-being and their ability to function in ordinary tasks of living. The removal of a process that limits the individual and therefore reduces their ability to function within our communities demonstrates some of the areas of concern for those with LD.

The concept of stigma associated to learning disability

Having a LD can lead to a degree of stigmatization. As a concept, Goffman (1963) argued that stigma arises during social interaction, concerned that the social identity of the individual may be 'spoiled', marking the individual deviant which renders them incapable of fulfilling the role required of social interaction. This notion of stigma can be either felt or enacted and can be applied to many groups within society and covers many areas of health and long-term conditions. In using Goffman's interpretation of stigma, practitioners are able to appreciate the negativity and 'deeply discrediting' attributes of stigma. Link and Phelan (2001: 367) provide more detail in their explanation by arguing that stigma exists 'when elements of labelling, stereotyping, separation, status loss and discrimination occur together in a power situation that allows them'.

The debate about social value and social exclusion is complex, and provides clear evidence to support the difficulties highlighted in the management of care. In order to promote inclusion, society has to view the individual in a particular way. The literature for social value is extensive and compelling. Graeber (2001) provides a platform for understanding social value and its application to sociological interruption. When these notions are transferred to the LD person with epilepsy, the following considerations may be made. If both LD and epilepsy are represented as issues that are of low social value then there are clearly problematic cultural issues in terms of service provision and delivery. The allocation of resources is a prime example of the difficulties encountered by this group. Commissioning is a method employed in the NHS to ensure fairer, efficient and effective use of resources and finances. Here is the initial example of social exclusion in the form of reciprocal exchange, this is where the individual exchanges one service for other services using their contributions to 'the human community' (Gouldner 1960) as a form of human capital. This concept of exchange has been developed and explored over the past four decades and continues to provide in-depth debate to date (Trivers 1985; Nowak and Sigmund 1998). Walzer (1981) and Byrne (1999) further suggest that this bargaining system is used to ascertain our value and what we contribute to our communities and therefore helps decide who we are, 'our value'.

Within LD this application to the argument provides the following question of moral obligation: how can a person with LD enter such a contract (Komter 1996)? The exchange of goods would suggest an ability to provide goods and, as previously noted, this is not always the case for those with LD. Graeber (2001) enables further conclusions to be drawn: if reciprocal exchange forms a part of communities, then it determines our social value and how we are judged. In Scenario 1 Richard had received good care during his hospitalization but his ongoing care had been poor and could be described as almost life threatening. Indeed examples of poor health can be seen in *Death by Indifference* (MENCAP 2007) where examples of poor service resulted in the death of people with LD and raised some unanswered questions. MENCAP provided data and examples of six deaths that occurred as a result of people with LD being seen as low priority. This demonstrated that many people with LD are at risk and being seen as low priority. The document also concluded that many health care professionals did not have a good understanding of LD which in turn meant that they did not involve or consult with clients, families or carers. Health care professionals rely inappropriately on their own estimates of quality of life. This meant that some of the examples provided within *Death by Indifference* make reference to the use of inappropriate language and thus excluding the person or their carer from being active participants in their own health care.

Stigma associated with epilepsy

It is often considered that people with LD and epilepsy have a 'double stigma'. Scambler (1989) and Scambler and Hopkins (1986) define stigma in epilepsy through a theoretical perspective: felt and enacted stigma. This theoretical view gives insight into how and why the individual with epilepsy may respond in certain ways. The stigmatization response to epilepsy is different to other areas of health: for some the secrecy embodies the stigma of the condition and provides a rationale for the changes and collaborations that are echoed in many of the relationships that surround epilepsy in particular groups. Link and Phelan (2001) argue that stigma can be conceptualized in diverse ways and that this is possible because stigma may be regarded as an entirely context-dependent notion. Scambler (1989) points out that although there have been great advances in both the understanding and treatment of epilepsy many of those with this disorder continue to be stigmatized by it. Stephen (Scenario 2) has the support of a multi-disciplinary team but his perception of epilepsy overshadows the support mechanisms that are in place.

Jacoby (2002) goes further, stating that the stigma of epilepsy can be linked to a number of factors, including under-resourced medical services, poor seizure control and inadequate knowledge of epilepsy. Neither informal stigma nor formal discrimination is inevitable for epilepsy patients; however, for many individuals, epilepsy remains a defining feature of their identity. Such issues are a source of considerable concern for a number of patients. In Jacoby et al. (2004) an opportunity to observe the level of public perceptions of stigma in the UK is provided and it is apparent that positive changes have occurred over the last three to four decades. However, when these changes are scrutinized they appear to be general, while individual cases still seem to have many of the attributes of felt stigma that have been evident for so many years. Having said that, the change in areas of quality of life and psychological well-being still causes difficulties for individuals. Overall, the study found that on the whole the population studied were well informed about epilepsy; this included the relationship to potential causes; the way in which seizures manifested themselves; and the way antiepileptic drugs were used to control seizure frequency. However, they found that those surveyed were less well informed about the causes of epilepsy, often considering an association with mental rather than physical conditions. A further but significant point was the finding that people with epilepsy are treated differently by society.

Scambler and Hopkins (1983) explored the perspective of people with epilepsy as a means of identifying how stigma can impact on quality of life. They found that the use of labelling results in the individual being 'a person with epilepsy' thereby ensuring stigmatization. The work of Goffman (1963) adds deeper understanding to the debate by highlighting 'the hiding of discreditable attributes'; acting as one who becomes socially withdrawn which develops difficulties enhanced by having epilepsy. Scambler and Hopkins debate the notion of felt and enacted stigma within epilepsy. The sociological notion of 'felt stigma' was more prevalent than 'enacted stigma'. This was encouraged by stigma coaches who helped keep epilepsy a secret, concealed the condition and added to the concept that it was bad. When coupled with LD this means that an individual with epilepsy may have an enormous amount of secrets. These secrets make the individual more vulnerable and indeed could exclude them from participating in everyday activities, relationships, jobs and life choices. It is these activities that ultimately determine our social value.

In Scenario 2, Stephen suffered 'felt stigma' as a result of his epilepsy which had a profound effect on his quality of life. He had seizures in the middle of activities he did not enjoy, especially when there was a crowd and no one had acknowledged him or when he felt he wanted to change the focus of the environment. It became obvious that seizures occurred when the greatest response was possible. The link between behaviour and seizure activity is an important one to practitioners. We can see the impact of epilepsy on Stephen who was coping with his learning disability, and although he had some degree of vulnerability he had overcome this in terms of his ability to function as an inclusive member of his community. The onset of epilepsy has meant changes to the way in which he now behaves and how he is viewed by others around him. Panayiotopoulos (2007) provided an explanation of behaviour and its links to generalized seizure types suggesting that impaired consciousness, as in epilepsy, can induce possible depression, agitation, hostility and aggression on occasions. Jacoby et al. (2005) debate a person's ability to interpret their environment and go some way to assist the practitioner in understanding and managing individual patterns of behaviour and provide ways to assist expression. It is agreed by many that side effects and behaviour are difficult to distinguish within LD. Koch-Stoecker (2002) and Kerr (2002) explain that many anti-epileptic drugs can exacerbate existing difficult behaviours and may induce or increase seizure activity within the individual. Koch-Stoecker states that there is an increased possibility of neurological disruption when antipsychotic medication is being used for behaviour management alongside anti-epileptic medication. When an individual has epilepsy and a LD it is also important to have an understanding of behaviour within LD and its link between communication and cognitive ability (Kerr 2004).

The difference between epilepsy and behaviour in LD is often difficult to establish but has an impact on care. This difficulty often causes some confusion in the diagnosis of epilepsy in LD, sometimes leading to misdiagnosis. To assist practitioners to differentiate, Kerr and Bowley (2001) and Kerr et al. (2009) highlight that within a seizure the behaviour is identical on each occasion but where there are issues of behaviour, there are variations to the particular behaviour. Scenario 2 (Stephen) illustrates the impact of epilepsy on an individual who was coping with his LD and, although with a degree of vulnerability, had overcome this in terms of his ability to function as an inclusive member of his community. The onset of epilepsy has meant changes to the way in which he now behaves and how he is viewed by others. The 'behaviour' (or acting out)

Seizure	Behaviour
◉ identical behaviour on each occasion	◉ variations in behaviour with circumstances
◉ no precipitating cause	◉ commonly precipitating causes
◉ unresponsive to communication or calming	

Figure 5.2 Offers some examples of differences between seizures and 'behaviours'.

acts as an indicator of his attempt to control his environment, something that could respond positively to calming and support. In recognizing the differences between epilepsy and behaviour, practitioners can successfully plan interventions and ensure plans reflect the needs presented. In addition, recognition of quality of life issues will help provide structure and appropriate care interventions (Baker 2001; Espie et al. 2001; Jacoby and Baker 2008).

Chapter summary

Quality of life is an important measurement of life satisfaction. The scenarios presented within this chapter have provided a platform to review some key issues pertaining to vulnerability within the area of LD and LD and epilepsy. Commonly used definitions and the incidences of both LD with epilepsy have been presented to set the scene for the reader and to give an indication of the essence of risk and vulnerability within LD. The first scenario highlights the vulnerability of a 57-year-old man living at home with his elderly mother and highlights the importance of individuals feeling secure within the community and being safe from harassment and harm. Scenario 1 also illustrates how the 'accessing' of appropriate health and social care can sometimes be less than straightforward but should be addressed by all agencies. Although stigma has been observed in Scenario 2 alongside epilepsy it is also evident to some extent in Scenario 1. The concept of stigma pervades LD as do equal access to services and all elements of normal living within the community. Similarly, the importance of empowerment and personalization apply to Stephen in Scenario 2. The second scenario emphasizes the incidence and impact of epilepsy on an individual with LD and epilepsy and introduces felt and enacted stigma. It also highlights how the behaviour of people can be changed in some way by epilepsy: this is especially so when the individual has a LD. Here again the impact on quality of life and the necessity to understand why an individual with LD responds in an adverse way to their lifestyle changes.

Notes

1   The chapter subscribes to the working definition of vulnerable adults provided by the Department of Health in 2004: 'a vulnerable adult must be 18 years or over and is, or may be in need of community care services by reason of mental or other disability, age or illness; further is, or may be unable to take care of him or herself, or is unable to protect him or herself from significant harm or serious exploitation'.

2   http://www.aboutlearningdisabilities.co.uk/social-inclusion-learning-disabilities.
     html.
3   NB: All Legislation pertaining to the rights of individuals apply equally to the
     LD population. These include Human Rights, Equality and Disabilities Legis-
     lation. The Mental Capacity Act (2005) because of its centrality to LD practice
     is concentrated within this the chapter.

References

Alborz, A., McNally, R. and Glendinning C. (2005). Access to health care for
    people with learning disabilities in the UK: mapping the issues and
    reviewing the evidence. *Journal of Health Services Research and Policy* 10:
    173–82.
All Party Parliamentary Group on Epilepsy (2007) *Wasted Money Wasted Lives.*
    London: Joint Epilepsy Council.
Baker, G. (2001) Assessment of quality of life in people with epilepsy: some
    practical implications. *Epilepsia*, 42(3): 66–9.
Beavis, J., Kerr, M. and Marson, A.G. (2007) *Non-pharmacological interventions for
    epilepsy in people with intellectual disabilities. Cochrane Database System*, 17(4).
Beran, R.G., Weber, S., Sungaran, R., Venn, N. and Hung, A. (2004) Review of the
    legal obligations of the doctor to discuss sudden unexplained death in epilepsy
    (SUDEP): a cohort controlled comparative cross matched study in an outpatient
    epilepsy clinic. *Seizure*, 13(7): 523–8.
Blume, W.T. et al. (2001) Glossary of descriptive terminology for ictal semiology:
    report of the International League Against Epilepsy Task Force on Classification
    and Terminology. *Epilepsia*, 42: 1212–18.
Brodie, M.J., Schachter, S.C. and Kwan, P. (2005) *Fast Facts: Epilepsy.* Oxford: Health
    Press.
Burchardt, T., Le Grand, J. and Piachaud, D. (2002) Introduction. In J. Hills, J. Le
    Grand and D. Piachaud (eds) *Understanding Social Exclusion.* Oxford: Oxford
    University Press.
Byrne, D. (1999) *Social Exclusion.* Buckingham: Open University Press.
Dempsey, I. and Foreman, P. (1997) Towards a clarification of empowerment as an
    outcome of disability service provision. *International Journal of Disability,
    Development and Education*, 44(4): 287–303.
Department of Health (DoH) (2001) *Valuing People: A New Strategy for Learning
    Disability for the 21st Century.* London: HMSO.
Department of Health (DoH) (2004) *Regulatory Impact Assessment: Protection of
    Vulnerable Adults.* London: HMSO.
Department of Health (2008) *Valuing People Now: From Progress to Transformation.*
    London: HMSO.

Emerson, E. and Hatton, C. (2004) *Estimating the Current Need/Demand for Supports for People with Learning Disabilities in England*. Lancaster: Institute for Health Research, Lancaster University.

Emerson, E. and Hatton, C. (2008) *People with Learning Disabilities in England*. Lancaster: Centre for Disability Research (CeDR), Lancaster University.

Epilepsy Action (2009) *Epilepsy in England: Time for Change*. Leeds: Epilepsy Action.

Espie, C.A., Watkins, J., Duncan, R. et al. (2001) Development and validation of the Glasgow Epilepsy Outcome Scale (GEOS): a new instrument for measuring concerns about epilepsy in people with mental retardation. *Epilepsia*, 42(8): 1043–51.

Espie, C.A., Watkins, J., Curtice, L. et al. (2003) Psychopathology in people with epilepsy and intellectual disability; an investigation of potential explanatory variables. *Journal of Neurological Neurosurgery Psychiatry*, 74: 1485–92.

Fisher, R.S., et al. (2005) Epileptic seizures and epilepsy: definitions proposed by the International League Against Epilepsy (ILAE) and the International Bureau for Epilepsy (IBE). *Epilepsia*, 46(4): 470–2.

Gaitatzis, A. and Sander, J.W. (2004) The mortality of epilepsy revisited. *Epileptic Disorders*, 6(1): 3–13.

Goffman, E. (1963) *Stigma: Notes on the Management of Spoiled Identity*. Englewood Cliffs, NJ: Prentice-Hall.

Gouldner, A.W. (1960), The norm of reciprocity: a preliminary statement. *American Sociological Review*, 25(2): 161–78.

Graeber, D. (2001) *Toward an Anthropological Theory of Value: The False Coin of Our Own Dreams*. New York: Palgrave.

Hitiris, N. et al. (2007) Mortality in epilepsy. *Epilepsy and Behaviour*, 10(3): 363–7.

International League Against Epilepsy/International Bureau for Epilepsy/World Health Organization (2003) *Global Campaign against Epilepsy: Out of the Shadows*. The Netherlands: International Bureau of Epilepsy.

Jacoby, A. (2002) Stigma, epilepsy, and quality of life. *Epilepsy and Behaviour*, 3(6): 10–20.

Jacoby, A. and Baker, G.A. (2008) Quality-of-life trajectories in epilepsy: a review of the literature. *Epilepsy Behaviour*, 12: 557–71.

Jacoby, A., Baker, G. and Snape, D. (2005) Epilepsy and social identity: the stigma of a chronic neurological disorder. *Lancet Neuro*, 4: 171–8.

Jacoby, A., Gorry, J., Gamble, C. and Baker, G.A. (2004) Public knowledge, private grief: a study of public attitudes to epilepsy in the United Kingdom and implications for stigma. *Epilepsia*, 45(11): 1405–15.

Joint Epilepsy Council (2005) *Epilepsy Prevalence, Incidence and other Statistics*. Leeds: Joint Epilepsy Council.

Kerr, M.P. (2002) Behavioral assessment in mentally retarded and developmentally disabled patients with epilepsy. *Epilepsy and Behaviour*, 3: S14–17.

Kerr, M.P. (2004) Improving the general health of people with learning disabilities. *Advances in Psychiatric Treatment*, 10: 200–206.

Kerr, M.P. and Bowley, C. (2001) Multidisciplinary and multiagency contributions to care for those with learning disability who have epilepsy. *Epilepsia*, 42: 55–6.

Kerr, M.P. and Wilcox, J. (2006) Epilepsy in people with learning disabilities. *Psychiatry*, 5(10): 372–7.

Kerr, M.P., Turky, A. and Huber, B. (2009) The psychosocial impact of epilepsy in adults with an intellectual disability. *Epilepsy Behaviour*, 15: S26–30.

Keywood, K., Fovargue, S. and Flynn, M. (1999). *Best Practice? Healthcare Decision-making by, with and for Adults with Learning Disabilities*. Manchester: NDT.

Koch-Stoecker, S. (2002) Antipsychotic drugs and epilepsy: indications and treatment guidelines. *Epilepsia*, 43: 19–24.

Komter, A.E. (1996) Reciprocity as a principle of exclusion: gift giving in The Netherlands. *Sociology*, 30(2): 299–316.

Lanfear, J. (2002) The individual with epilepsy. *Nursing Standard*, 16: 43–53.

Leplège, A. and Hunt, S. (1997) The problem of quality of life in medicine. *Journal of the American Medical Association*, 278(1): 47–50.

Lhatoo, S.D. and Sander, J.W.A.S. (2001) The epidemiology of epilepsy and learning disability. *Epilepsia*, 42, Supplement 1: 6–9.

Link, B.G. and Phelan, J.C. (2001) Conceptualizing stigma. *Annual Review of Sociology*, 27: 363–85.

Loughran, S.J. and O'Brien, D. (2001) Health care, epilepsy and learning disabilities. *Nursing Standard*, 15(22): 33–4.

Mason, T., Carlisle, C., Watkins, C. and Whitehead, E. (eds) (2001) *Stigma and Social Exclusion in Health Care*. London: Routledge.

Matthews, T. et al. (2008) A general practice based prevalence study of epilepsy among adults with intellectual disabilities and of its association with psychiatric disorders. Behaviour disturbance and carer stress. *Journal of Intellectual Disability Research*, 52: 163–73.

MENCAP (2000) *Living in Fear*. London: MENCAP.

MENCAP (2004) *Treat Me Right*. London: MENCAP.

MENCAP (2007) *Death by Indifference*. London: MENCAP.

Michael, J. and Richardson, A. (2008) *Healthcare for All: Report of the Independent Inquiry into Access to Healthcare for People with Learning Disabilities*. London: Department of Health.

Morton, B., Richardson, A. and Duncan, S. (2006) Sudden unexpected death in epilepsy (SUDEP): don't ask, don't tell? *Journal of Neurology, Neurosurgery & Psychiatry*, 77(2): 199–202.

Nashef, L. (1997) SUDEP: terminology and definitions. *Epilepsia*, 38(11): 56–8.

National Institute of Clinical Excellence (NICE) (2004) *Quick Reference Guide: The Epilepsies – Diagnosis and Management of the Epilepsies in Adults in Primary and Secondary Care*. London: NICE.

National Institute of Clinical Excellence (NICE) (2010–11) *Quality and Outcomes Framework (QOF) Indicator Development Programme*. London: NICE.

Nowak, M.A. and Sigmund, K. (1998) Evolution of indirect reciprocity by image scoring. *Nature*, 393: 573–7.

Panayiotopoulos, C.P. (2007) *A Clinical Guide io Epileptic Syndromes and Their Treatment*. London: Springer.

Scambler, G. (1983) Being epileptic: sociology of stigmatizing condition. Unpublished PhD thesis, University of London.

Scambler, G. (1989) *Epilepsy*. London: Tavistock.

Scambler, G. and Hopkins, A. (1986) Being epileptic: coming to terms with stigma. *Sociology of Health & Illness*, 8(1): 26–43.

Scope (2008) *Getting Away with Murder: Disabled People's Experiences of Hate Crime in the UK*. London: Scope.

Tompson, T., Walczak, T., Sillanpaa, M. and Sander, J.W. (2005) Sudden unexpected death in epilepsy: a review of incidence and risk factors. *Epilepsia*, 46(11): 54–61.

Trivers, R. (1985) *Social Evolution*. Menlo Park, CA: Benjamin/Cummings.

Walzer, M. (1981) The distribution of membership. In P.G. Brown and H. Shue (eds) *Boundaries, National Autonomy and Its Limits*. Totowa, NJ: Rowman and Littlefield.

Wong, J.G., Clare, I.C.H., Holland, A.J., Watson, P.C. and Gunn, M. (2002) The capacity of people with a 'mental disability' to make a health care decision. *Psychological Medicine*, 30: 295–306.

World Health Organization (2001) *International Classification of Functioning Disability and Health: ICF*. Geneva: WHO.

Other sources

www.epilepsy.org.uk/info/whatisepilepsy.html

www.jointepilepsycouncil.org.uk/About-Epilepsy.html

www.touchneurology.com/articles/epilepsy-care-whoilaeibe-global-campaign-against-epilepsy

www.who.int/mediacentre/factsheets/fs999/en/index.html

6   Insecure accommodation

Margaret Greenfields

Lack of a secure place to live is by definition a marker of vulnerability, exposing indi-viduals of all ages to a wide range of risks. The fundamental need for a safe place to dwell has been recognized in policy discourse since mid-19th-century reformers cham-pioned the need to provide people with decent living conditions as a first step towards access to employment, health and social integration. Homelessness and insecure accommodation encompass far more than 'rough sleeping', and this chapter explores the experiences and risks of exclusion (and routes into and out of homelessness) for individuals at different stages of their lives. Particular reference is paid to the intersec-tionality of risk associated with personal characteristics such as gender, age, sexual orientation and disability as well as consideration of 'exacerbating' risk factors for homelessness or being insecurely accommodated.

Learning objectives

Readers of this chapter will be able to:

- understand the concept of insecure accommodation and the multi-factorial risks associated with this status;
- demonstrate awareness of the interplay of factors which expose individuals to homelessness and insecure accommodation at different life stages;
- describe the impact of discrimination and structural barriers which exacer-bate difficulties for people experiencing insecure accommodation;
- identify good practice initiatives and partnership opportunities for engaging with marginalized homeless and insecurely accommodated people.

The demand for affordable and high-quality accommodation is vastly outstripped by supply, particularly in areas of high employment where in-migration (both internal and from abroad) creates a significant pressure on access to housing and enables some unscrupulous landlords to maximize profits by exploiting tenants through the provision of sub-standard and over-crowded accommodation (see further Chapter 12 on housing problems faced by migrant workers), which breach both tenancy protection and health and safety regulations. Poor-quality or over-crowded housing are implicated in the exacerbated risk factors facing the homeless and insecurely accommodated and residence in such properties may act as a proxy marker for identifying those at risk of homelessness, especially when such tenants are members of excluded groups such as marginalized minority ethnic communities (Garvie 2004; Office of the Deputy Prime Minister (ODPM) 2005; Phillips 2008), migrant workers (Shelter Cmyru 2010) or young people who have left care and who have no family support network (Coombes 2004).

Yet despite the large number and variety of people who are living in insecure accommodation, certain stereotypes prevail in relation to the 'type' of person who is homeless – with a typical conception being that of a young male with substance use issues (often with a dog 'on a string') or an unwashed elderly man with mental health problems living in a doorway surrounded by his meagre possessions in bags. Yet the belief that homeless people have deliberately excluded themselves from society is belied by evidence showing that homelessness is caused by a complex interplay between a person's individual circumstances and adverse 'structural' factors outside their control (Ravenhill 2000; Shelter 2007). While for some people a sudden crisis can lead to homelessness or residence in insecure accommodation, for the majority, a sequence of difficulties builds up over years until a crisis occurs. Accordingly, strategies to engage with individuals who are vulnerable to homelessness and effective models to address the issue require both a clear comprehension of causative factors (and appropriate interventions) and awareness of the implications of multi-factorial vulnerability across the life span.

Counting the homeless population

It is difficult to estimate the total numbers of homeless people because of the fluctuating nature of the homeless population. Various forms of homelessness (e.g. 'street homeless' and those on waiting lists for accommodation but who might be 'sofa surfing' and living with relatives or friends) are counted in different ways by various agencies and government departments.

A number of datasets are available which attempt to provide information on the homeless population: some statistics are snapshot figures that count numbers of people at a particular moment in time while others are 'flow' data which count people becoming homeless over a period of time.

Homeless Link (the national charity which supports people and organizations working directly with homeless people in England) has a website which contains a number of resources including annual reports and briefings. The page on 'facts and figures' in relation to homelessness is available at: www.homeless.org.uk/facts.

Definitions and types of homelessness and insecure accommodation

While a colloquial definition of homelessness will tend towards the assumption of a 'rough sleeper', the legal definition of someone who is homeless is in fact wider, encompassing both those without a roof over their heads and individuals who do not have a place which they have a legal entitlement to occupy (thus including people 'staying' with family members or friends, squatters, and Gypsies and Travellers who are not resident on an authorized site: see further Chapter 11 for a discussion on Gypsy and Traveller site issues). See Table 6.1 for types of 'homelessness' and insecure accommodation.

Table 6.1 Types of 'homelessness' and insecure accommodation

Roofless	Rough sleepers
Houseless	Hostels/shelters
	Bed and Breakfast accommodation
	Living in a car/van or boat (not specifically adapted or non-residential accommodation)
Insecure	Institutions (hospitals, or prisons or in care)
Accommodation	Squats
	Living as a temporary guest
	Facing eviction as a result of mortgage or rent arrears *or* from short-term accommodation (including those living in friends/ relatives' homes, or short-term rented property, or where living under a 'licence' with no security of tenure)
	'Tied accommodation' linked to remaining in a particular employment (see further Chapter 12)
	Gypsy site without planning permission (including on the 'roadside'; see further Chapter 11)

(Continued)

Table 6.1 (*Continued*)

	Experiencing threats/intimidation from landlord or other tenants so unable to remain living in present accommodation (personal safety at risk)
	Severely sub-standard accommodation (e.g. illegal housing in multiple occupation (HMO) or poorly maintained property with leaking roof, dangerous wiring, etc.; see further Chapter 12 for a discussion on migrant workers' living arrangements)
'Hidden homeless'	Unable to establish separate place of residence and not feasible to remain in current situation (e.g. severely over-crowded while living/staying with parents, family or friends on a rent-free basis)
	'Sofa-surfing' between a number of residences
Lodgings	Private rented (sharing premises with landlord)
	Communal lodging house (see further Chapter 12 in relation to migrant workers)

Source: Table adapted and developed from Smith (2003) and New Policy Institute/Crisis (2004).

The causes of homelessness

The causes of homelessness and residence in insecure accommodation are many. Similarly, the risk factors faced by individuals are dependent upon the 'type' of homelessness they are experiencing ('street' homelessness being merely the tip of the iceberg in terms of those who do not have access to a secure place to live) and also vary as a result of personal circumstances and the intersectionality of vulnerabilities which may occur so that, for example, a disabled woman with mental health problems living in a squat is at greater risk than a young couple or single man without health difficulties living with relatives in an over-crowded flat. However, regardless of the individual characteristics which may exacerbate the dangers to a person, leading vulnerability to crystallize into risk of harm, the primary reasons for homeless can be classified as follows:

- *Family conflict/relationship breakdown* and being asked to leave the family home (which can include parental/child conflict, fleeing domestic violence or relationship breakdown). This overall category was cited as the main cause of their homelessness by 69 per cent of rough sleeper respondents in a 2007 Shelter report. Ravenhill (2000) found that for all homeless and insecurely accommodated people, 'inter-personal/family conflict' was the most common reason given for their housing status, regardless of age or gender.

- *Domestic violence:* Lakhani and Merrick (2008) report that 20 per cent of women who are homeless (whether living in hostels, 'hidden homeless' staying with friends, or sleeping rough) are victims of domestic violence who have left accommodation in search of a place of safety.

- *Substance use/abuse* issues were implicated in homelessness for 30 per cent of rough sleepers interviewed by Shelter in 2007. Family or relationship breakdown which leads to homelessness may also result from substance abuse (e.g. where alcohol use is associated with domestic violence or youth cannabis or polydrug use ends in parents requesting that the young person leaves home). Loss of employment and disability issues associated with problem substance use may also lead to a cycle of homelessness and insecure accommodation (see further Chapter 9 for a case study of multiple exclusions). A 2002 study on behalf of the Home Office and Department of Health reported that homelessness and substance misuse were often closely linked, finding that around 75 per cent of single homeless people were misusing drugs (Randall and Drugscope 2002).

- *Institutionalization:* one in four rough sleepers were found to have left prison and had nowhere to go, many having lost their homes while 'inside' and having no family or friends who would provide them with accommodation (Shelter 2007). People leaving institutional settings (e.g. the armed forces, prison or care leavers) are particularly vulnerable to homelessness. Not only may their previous life experiences and complex personal histories mean that they are not equipped with appropriate budgeting or coping skills to manage independent living, but they may also have a range of other needs (e.g. mental health issues, post-traumatic stress disorder, literacy and numeracy problems), disrupted community attachments and lack of familiarity with anything other than an institutional setting where their daily needs such as accommodation, food and so on are met for them. Data from a telephone survey of homelessness projects and specialist advice centres in England and Wales (Homeless Link 2009) found that 18 per cent of clients were prison leavers, 14 per cent of clients were care leavers and 6 per cent of clients were ex-service personnel.

- *Mental health issues:* 19 per cent of rough sleepers (Shelter 2007) reported having mental health problems, although whether they had become homeless as a result of their health needs or their homelessness exacerbated their condition was unclear (see further Chapter 4 and Case Study at Chapter 9).

- *Insecure accommodation* (which in many cases blends into homelessness) while regarded as a less precarious situation than 'statutory homelessness' tends to be commonly associated less with 'personal deficit' models than with poverty and lack of affordable housing. Accordingly, many insecurely accommodated individuals and families have either been made redundant in a precarious economic climate or are the 'working poor' who may be unable to access secure tenancies at an affordable rent, or who cannot afford to buy property and thus have found themselves dependent on relatives and friends, squatting in empty buildings, sharing over-crowded accommodation or living in hostels or property 'tied' to their employment (Penny 2010).

Learning exercise

Imagine a situation where you found yourself at crisis point: you are being made redundant and don't have enough savings to pay your rent for the six weeks which you have been told it will take for Local Housing Allowance (LHA) to 'come through'. Your (private rented) landlord tells you that he only wants working people – you will have to pay your rent in advance until your LHA is sorted out if you want to stay and, anyway, if you don't find a job within three months he will let your flat to someone else. Meanwhile your credit card bill has arrived, you have an overdraft at your bank which you can pay off by using most of your last salary payment but you have another six months left on your mobile phone contract and your phone payment is due. You are 21 years old and have lived independently for three years but have just discovered that your social security benefit entitlements (which take a few weeks to be assessed) are lower than for someone 'over 25'.

What would you do?

Risks associated with homelessness

While some risks and disadvantages remain constant across the life-span for insecurely accommodated and homeless people (e.g that of experiencing theft of belongings or being a victim of violence for those sleeping rough), the cumulative impact of these factors and the likelihood of experiencing a particular type of harm will also depend upon a synergy of existing protective elements and the resilience of an individual (state of health, access to a range of capitals, protective factors which limit likelihood of mental ill-health, etc.), personal characteristics such as age, disability and ethnicity and the duration (and type) of poor accommodation experienced. While specific characteristic-related risks (e.g. associated with being an older homeless person) are considered below, core problematic issues, common to homeless or insecurely accommodated people can be classified as follows.

Personal safety

Rough sleepers are at greatly exacerbated risk of violent assault than are surrounding populations (including those insecurely accommodated in hostels and squats). The dangers to rough sleepers include violence from other 'street homeless' people – particularly associated with use of alcohol and drugs or those having an episode of mental ill-health, and also from passing members of the public who may themselves be drunk or simply regard homeless vulnerable people with abhorrence. Ramesh (2010) cites the Director of a London homelessness charity as reporting that rough sleepers 'ended up in A&E five times more often than a regular citizen and were 15 times more likely to be a victim of violence'. A number of well-publicized court cases and newspaper reports in Britain over the past decade have presented horrific evidence of rough sleepers being attacked, and in some cases murdered, by gangs of young men, often after the attackers have spent the night drinking.[1] For women in particular, the dangers of sexual assault both from other rough sleepers and passers-by add a further dimension to the risks of homelessness.

Other insecurely accommodated people, while not at such great risk as street sleepers, may also find themselves exposed to violence and threats to their personal safety when making use of hostels, Bed and Breakfast accommodation or residing in shared housing (e.g. those provided for migrant workers). Agencies working with homeless people note that many homeless people avoid using shelter services other than in times of dire emergency or when the weather is extremely cold, as they fear that their personal safety may be compromised. While shelters do their best to protect residents, of necessity, most shelters are run with 'skeleton staffing' levels, often supported by a high percentage of volunteers who may not be familiar with dealing with violent or aggressive behaviour. Accordingly, personal safety cannot be guaranteed for those using the facilities. Residents who are typically expected to share rooms or dormitories often find themselves living alongside violent offenders, substance addicts and people with mental health problems. Shelter (2007) reported that over half of shelter users they interviewed reported problems with other service users relating to drugs and alcohol, violence, theft, bullying, noise and general arguments. Although Bed and Breakfast accommodation and multiple-occupancy housing shared with strangers may not offer quite such a high degree of risk, the use of shared cooking and bathroom facilities and typically poor security precautions such as a simple 'yale' lock on bedroom doors or small bolt on bathrooms and toilets can expose residents to risk of theft, and physical and sexual assault from chaotic or substance misusing co-residents.

Access to health care

For both street homeless and insecurely accommodated people, access to health care and appropriate medical treatment can be problematic. 'Street homeless' or rough sleepers are unsurprisingly the most vulnerable group, with an average life expectancy of 42 (Crisis 1996) and a death rate (for rough sleepers aged between 45 and 62) 25 times that of people of the same age group in the general population (Bines 1994). For the most vulnerable homeless people their accommodation status multiplies the risk factors for poor health. The Queens Nursing Institute (2007) report that rough sleeping makes it difficult for people to achieve even basic health and well-being as a result of poor nutrition (e.g. reliance on 'fast food' and infrequent meals or eating out-of-date food thrown out by shops), difficulties accessing hygiene facilities, preoccupations with personal safety and lack of privacy, warmth, space and access to warm clothing.

For many insecurely accommodated people, anxiety associated with their homelessness can trigger mental health problems for the first time or exacerbate issues which already exist (see further Chapter 4). Bines (1994) found that mental health problems were 8 times higher for hostel and Bed and Breakfast residents and 11 times higher among people sleeping rough than among the general population, and that for people who sleep rough there is a 35 times greater risk of suicide across all age ranges than is found among the general population (Crisis 1996). Poor health behaviours such as excessive use of alcohol and other substances with a potential to be abused (including long-term use of prescription drugs for depression and associated conditions), coupled with very high rates of cigarette smoking, are commonly found among homeless and insecurely accommodated individuals. Anecdotally, homelessness service users report that they are often less concerned with their long-term health than in finding a way to overcome their daily circumstances, thus the immediate and pleasurable impact of smoking a cigarette or drinking alcohol appears of more import than the potential that they will shorten their life by continuing such activities (Health Development Agency 2004).

Even for those insecurely accommodated people living with relatives or friends, anxiety, depression and associated ill-health can have a markedly negative impact on well-being and self-care. In 2003 Crisis estimated that of the 400,000 'hidden homeless' in Britain living with family, on friends' floors, squats, hostels or Bed and Breakfasts 1 in 3 had mental health problems, 1 in 4 had a drug addiction and one-fifth were alcoholics (Frith 2003). Difficulties in sharing of space and access to kitchen areas means that for people living in hostels, shared housing or even in relatives and friends' homes, their health can potentially suffer through lack of opportunity to cook nutritious meals. For older people, those with pre-existing health issues or families with dependent children who are more vulnerable to the impacts of poor diet and who are in any case more likely to be living on a smaller, fixed income than working 'hidden homeless', the long-term effects on their health of lack of freshly cooked, good quality food may include exacerbation of depressive illnesses, malnutrition and increased risk of contracting infections. Residence in poor-quality and overcrowded accommodation is also significantly implicated in rates of tuberculosis (TB), respiratory conditions such as asthma, the contraction of infectious skin diseases and an enhanced risk of lifelong poor health for children and young people growing up in such conditions (ODPM 2004).

Obtaining medical treatment for health conditions (where the individual identifies that a need is great enough to seek medical care[2]) for both rough sleepers and the insecurely accommodated can also be difficult. Both primary care and specialist mental health services may be reluctant to take on the care of people who are homeless or living in insecure accommodation. The Queens Nursing Institute (2007) reported that homeless people are 40 times less likely to be registered with a GP than are those with a stable place to live.

Bed and Breakfast residents or people living in squats or multiple occupancy housing with high mobility of tenants, often find that local medical practices will only accept them as 'temporary patients', which minimizes the likelihood of them being able to access preventative treatment or specialist care such as referrals to counsellors or other psychological services.

Rough sleepers in particular are only likely to be able to access medical support when it is made available through drop-in clinics or at hostels or if their health is poor enough for them to need to attend an A&E clinic at a hospital. Given the prevalence of mental health needs among homeless people, this group is severely excluded in terms of access to appropriate mental health services which are typically organized on a geographical or GP practice list

---

Good practice example

A cross-borough practitioner-led health outreach programme operates across the London Boroughs of Lambeth, Southwark and Lewisham. The '3 Boroughs Homelessness Team' service runs drop-in clinics attached to hostels and day centres across the area. The clinics are nurse-led but also employ sessional GPs, chiropodists and a dentist.

The service offers one-to-one health screening, health promotion advice and referrals to more specialist services such as psychiatric teams as well as supporting group health-related activities. They also provide advice on hospital discharge, run user involvement health projects and facilitate IT development for service users and front-line homelessness staff. The team members include a trainer who provides specialist courses on health-related matters for homelessness centre workers as well as a nurse practitioner specializing in youth homelessness.

A key strength of the service is the facilitation of health promotion activities and referrals in partnership with hostel staff and members of the agencies who are involved in front-line service provision for homeless and insecurely accommodated people.

Public health functions/project initiated by the service include:

- vaccination clinics at hostels and day centres offering Hepatitis A and B, Meningitis C and Influenza vaccines;
- an audit of asthma care services received by homeless people;
- chlamydia and syphilis screening services (of particular importance for homeless people who may intermittently engage with sex work or trade sexual activities for a warm place to stay), emergency contraception, the provision of condoms and 'safer sex' advice assistance with GP registration;
- minor illness and minor injury assessment and management;
- the provision of certain 'immediately necessary' medications; (e.g. antibiotics, asthma inhalers, etc.).
- the triage of acute physical and mental health conditions, and referral into A&E and secondary care as necessary;
- wound care (including leg ulcer management);
- assistance with TB screening programmes;
- referral to drug, alcohol and other specialist services;
- smoking cessation support.

basis. Accordingly, if a homeless person is not registered with a local GP, they are likely to be perceived as being 'mobile' and thus not the responsibility of any particular mental health team. Where homeless people are hospitalized for either physical or mental health needs, on discharge, further barriers may exist to accessing accommodation or ongoing medical support, particularly if local authorities refuse to accept an individual as being in priority need of housing or considers that they do not have an long-term connection to a local area and thus are not eligible for accommodation.

Continuity of healthcare is thus frequently disrupted for both homeless and insecurely accommodated people as services are generally designed to meet the needs of longer-established residents who can establish an ongoing relationship with their health care providers. Best practice for engaging with the diverse and complex health needs of homeless and insecurely accommodated people is therefore likely to involve a combination of targeted and opportunistic health interventions which enable individuals to access health services while in a 'safe' environment which they are already attending to obtain support for other homeless related issues such as benefits advice or information on housing rights.

Education, training and employment

While some insecurely accommodated people (e.g. those living in 'tied accom-modation' or with relatives) are engaged in employment, training and educa-tion, for probably the majority of homeless people the stress and insecurity of their circumstances precludes access to (or retention of) employment and education. Homeless children (including those living in over-crowded and insecure accommodation), while required by law to be enrolled in schools, frequently experience volatility of movement with inevitable impacts on their educational opportunities.

Families residing in low-cost houses in multiple occupancy, or privately rented rooms, and asylum seekers facing dispersal and removal to other locali-ties may be expected to change their children's schools frequently as they are required to move at short notice (Stanley 2002; Harker 2006). It has been calcu-lated that a high percentage of families claiming local housing allowance are affected by the decrease in finances available to support low-income or work-less households' rental costs (announced June 2010, with effect from April 2011) and inevitably this will result in a movement away from certain higher cost localities for households claiming this allowance or indeed increase over-crowding as people move into smaller, cheaper accommodation (O'Grady 2010). Indeed for many children and young people, frequent movement between educational establishments is dependent upon the type of accommo-dation they occupy and their homelessness status, for example whether resi-dent in local authority-supplied Bed and Breakfast or hostel accommodation which may even be provided out of their 'home' area to make fiscal savings. On each move, not only do children and young people experience disruption of friendships and have to engage with different teaching strategies or educa-tional syllabi, but often they find themselves in circumstances with limited or inappropriately noisy or crowded spaces in which to study perhaps because their entire family are living in a single room. Significant evidence exists that children from homeless households are more likely to suffer from bullying, unhappiness and stigmatization in schools (Harker 2006) as well as achieve exam results at a significantly lower standard than their peers in less crowded, better quality housing (Morris and Easton 2008).

Social isolation/stigma

Homeless and insecurely accommodated people frequently report feeling stig-matized in relation to their housing situation. While rough sleepers are the most obviously excluded group of homeless people – and are frequently exposed to verbal and sometimes physical abuse (often related to erroneous presumptions about their characters, personal circumstances and individual deficits which *must* have led to their housing situation) – research and anecdotal reports from front-line staff suggests that the overwhelming majority of insecurely housed and homeless people report feelings of shame and personal failure (Casey et al. 2007; Department for Social Development Northern Ireland (DSDNI) 2007; Williams 2010).

For children and families living in hostel accommodation or privately rented rooms the fact that they typically have inadequate space to enable them to invite friends from school to come home to play or eat dinner inevitably places them 'outside' of peer groups, and precludes numerous social activities. Similarly, young people who are living with relatives or friends in concealed (over-crowded) households or who are sofa-surfing report that their social lives must generally take place away from where they are living as a way of avoiding conflict with the householder with whom they are staying. The impact of being unable to return hospitality or to be able to enter into adult networks and relationships will often cause withdrawal from social circles or a tendency only to engage with people in similar circumstances who will 'understand' their homelessness experience.

Older people who have become homeless or insecurely housed (perhaps living with relatives on a temporary basis or in rented rooms or hostel accommodation after discharge from hospital) after having had their own home, report finding the social isolation and lack of privacy particularly difficult to cope with, marking them out as having failed to achieve the stability which is 'expected' of older people. The fact that older people are more likely to spend time at 'home' as they age, can particularly emphasize their dependency upon others, minimize their opportunities to develop independent external activities and increase their sense of social isolation (Pannell 2005).

The responses to social isolation practised by many homeless people appear to conform to Goffman's (1968) theoretical model of stigma management, in particular, 'passing' by concealing their housing status to new acquaintances until it becomes no longer possible to do so, or withdrawing into a stigmatized group and disengaging from 'mainstream society' and thus perpetuating the concept of 'difference' between housed community members and those who have no secure place to live.

Individuals and families who are accepted as in priority need of housing and who are placed in temporary accommodation (e.g. asylum seekers or newly housed Gypsies and Travellers) also report that social isolation can result from being rehoused away from their local area (perhaps as a local authority cost-saving exercise) or in a geographical location where they are isolated from their culture and community. Young people anecdotally report fear of falling foul of local gangs if they are moved from one locality to another where they have no connections and little idea of the interplay of area loyalties. For all insecurely accommodated households or frequent movers (including those who are temporarily living with close relatives or friends where 'internal' household tensions may also occur), support networks are at risk of becoming strained at a period of time when people are at their most vulnerable. Where access to educational and health services becomes disrupted the impacts of loss of such vital connections can further deepen social exclusion and isolation.

Personal characteristics and the domains of risk

In addition to the generic risks posed by homelessness or insecure accommodation, certain groups face particular difficulties or an increased risk of homelessness as a result of society's response to their personal characteristics (e.g. disability, age, ethnicity, sexual orientation and gender). To some extent homelessness legislation takes account of these 'protected characteristics' by recognizing that when an inter-sectionality of vulnerabilities occurs an individual is at greatly increased risk. Accordingly they are likely to be recognized as in 'priority need' of housing. Thus someone without dependent children who is disabled and at risk of homelessness as a result of experiencing violence targeted on their sexual orientation or race is more likely to be able to access accommodation provided by a registered social landlord (RSL) than a single person without additional needs. However, despite the security offered to particularly vulnerable individuals by access to RSL properties, considerable risks still exist, as the very nature of these protected characteristics means that an individual may potentially experience prejudice or hostility from surrounding tenants once rehoused (e.g. racist discrimination or harassment associated with mental illness) and learning disabilities are still major problems in many localities.[3]

The following summary of factors which expose individuals or groups to particular risk of harm are based upon the domains which fall within the remit of the Equality Act 2010 and which are of specific policy concern to the Equality and Human Rights Commission.

Gender

While women are more likely than men to be the sole carers of children, and thus a proportionately greater number of homeless or insecurely housed women may be accepted as being in priority need by local authorities, patterns of homeless vary significantly by gender. Women are more likely to be 'hidden homeless' than are men and have largely remained invisible in policy discourse until relatively recently. Crisis (2006) reported that 11 per cent of rough sleepers in London were women, although this was likely to be an undercount, given women's tendency to seek to sleep in 'hidden' locations such as locked car parks or in relatively isolated areas to avoid sexual harassment and abuse. Homeless women are reported to be particularly vulnerable to mental illness, often as a result of experiences of domestic and sexual abuse (Crisis 2009) and frequently to have experienced high levels of trauma prior to becoming homeless. In response to their homelessness an 'alarming number' of homeless or insecurely accommodated women engaged in 'unwanted sexual liaisons' to secure somewhere to live, resorted to prostitution or returned to abusive partners rather than sleep rough. Domestic violence is implicated in at least 20 per cent of cases of female homelessness (Lakhani and Merrick 2008) and in many cases of youth homelessness young women report sexual violence or bullying by family members as a trigger for leaving home.

Single men report high levels of homelessness following the breakdown of relationships or after leaving institutional care or the armed forces. Males without significant qualifying characteristics (e.g disability) are extremely unlikely to be regarded as in priority need of housing as they are unlikely to be carers of children (Scottish Executive Central Research Unit (SECRU) 2002). Accordingly, single homeless men are particularly likely to become street homeless or to live in squats. A significant percentage of single homeless men become long-term residents of B&B hostels or reside in bed-sits or other shared accommodation (Homeless Link 2009).

Age

Significant research exists into the causes of youth homelessness (e.g. Quilgars et al. 2008) which consistently finds that family conflict in teenage years is the leading cause of young people leaving home. For many young people leaving home and becoming insecurely accommodated or homeless is the culmination of a number of years of tension and domestic problems. A significant number of young people become homeless following arguments with parents about substance use or addiction and/or offending behaviours (Wincup et al. 2003).

Homelessness projects statistics indicate that a high percentage of young service users have been 'looked after children' or former unaccompanied asylum seekers (Homeless Link 2009) who have experienced a traumatic life history, often have no family support and typically low life skills and educational attainment on leaving care, exposing them to a high risk of homelessness or unstable accommodation history (Centrepoint 2006). Significant evidence exists to suggest that young care leavers are at particular risk of entering into a rapid downward spiral which may include early parenthood, involvement with the criminal justice system, substance abuse, entering into unstable, abusive or violent relationships and the associated loss of tenancies or housing placements (Stein 2006).

At the opposite end of the life cycle, and contrary to the common perception that as people age they are more likely to remain living at a single location, research evidence suggests that increasing numbers of older people are becoming homeless or insecurely housed.

The reasons why older people become homeless do not vary particularly from those of other age groups, although unsurprisingly, a very low percentage of older people are rough sleepers with the majority being 'hidden homeless'. Many people within the older age groups have, prior to their experience of insecure accommodation, lived in stable housing and do not have any underlying vulnerability such as substance use or mental health issues. Accordingly, older homeless people are less likely to have been in contact with statutory services prior to becoming insecurely accommodated and may feel constrained from seeking preventative advice by a sense of shame or a belief that homelessness results from personal deficits.

Scenario for reflection

Are older people often 'invisible' to service providers because of stereotypes and assumptions relating to homeless people? Are agencies more likely to concentrate on working with 'high-visibility' groups or individuals who actively seek information? Reflect on what methods might be most effective in engaging with and providing appropriate information to older isolated people who may be at risk of homelessness. Do existing consultation methods (e.g. via internet which may not be available to many older people; through written materials which may be problematic for individuals with literacy challenges or who do not speak or read English as a first language; or by requiring a person to attend an office in person which may prove hard for someone with physical or mental health needs) provide the most appropriate way of disseminating information? How much does your 'quick' response to these questions reflect your own generational or socio-economic/cultural background?

Race/ethnicity

The rates of homelessness among different ethnic groups varies significantly across Britain with black and minority ethnic (BME) service users in rural localities represented at far lower levels than the rate at which they are found nationally. In areas of high urban density which have long-established BME communities and historical patterns of in-migration (e.g. London, Manchester, Liverpool) BME populations make up a relatively large percentage of the local community and are accordingly represented in homelessness statistics at higher rates. A danger exists, however, in assuming that members of all BME populations experience homelessness (and types of tenure associated with homelessness/rates of over-crowding) at a similar level. Such a simplistic analysis ignores the socio-economic variables between distinct BME communities as educational attainment, average family size and typical patterns of employment will all provide protective factors against homelessness or insecure accommodation. Despite the variables which exist (e.g. Asian and Chinese people are less likely to access homelessness services than are Black Caribbean or Black African households), overall the 'ethnic penalty' associated with membership of a BME community greatly exacerbates the risk of becoming homeless or living in insecure accommodation. The housing-related exclusion experienced by Britain's BME populations is linked to a disproportionate concentration of BME communities in the poorest urban (typically inner city) locations, a tendency for members of these populations to be workless or living in poverty, and resident in the most deprived and over-crowded housing in the country.

A 2003 government-commissioned review of the evidence base on BME populations and housing (ODPM 2003) found that BME applicants equated to 22 per cent of households accepted as being statutory homeless by local authorities. On that basis BME people were at that time three times more likely to become homeless than white British people. Research commissioned to explore the high over-representation of BME households in homelessness statistics (ODPM 2005) reported that variations in routes into homelessness occurred for different communities. Domestic/family violence was found to be the leading cause of homelessness applications for both single Asian women and married women with dependent children, while Asian couples with children were more likely to report loss of a private rented tenancy or severe over-crowding/residence in dangerous premises. The under-representation of Asian applicants in statutory housing statistics suggested reliance on 'self-help' solutions to insecure accommodation or greater acceptance of sub-standard or over-crowded accommodation.

Black Caribbean applicants were found to be the most over-represented of BME communities in homelessness statistics. Typically, applications were made by long female-headed households, with family disputes occurring when a woman became pregnant and family or friends were no longer able or willing to accommodate her, although some degree of over-representation was found among single applicants suffering from mental illness and found to be in priority need.

In the analytical period covered by the ODPM report (2005) the Black African community was still relatively small (having more than doubled in London in the first decade of the 21st century and by 2007 accounting for 10.5 per cent of the BME population in Britain; see further Steele and Ahmed 2007), making it somewhat difficult to generalize trends in homelessness. However, review of the data supported suggestions that young people seeking accommodation were often in dispute with family members over cultural values, and that older people were often responding to the needs of family and friends who were no longer able to accommodate relatively newly arrived households which caused significant over-crowding in living conditions. A study on behalf of the London Borough of Islington (Steele and Ahmed 2007) found that reasons for homelessness among Black African households were predominantly caused by parents, relatives or friends asking other household members to leave following pregnancy, relationship breakdown and over-crowding. Pregnancy was found to be a common reason for seeking housing for Black African women who were 'established' in England and was typically associated with lone parenthood. Family breakdown (often involving domestic violence) was linked to greater independence for women and a lessening of cultural, community and hierarchical ties which created an expectation of male predominance.

Garvie (2004) reported a particularly sharp rise in homelessness applications from BME households between 1997 and 2004, explicitly linking this to the impacts of the recession occurring at that time. Further exacerbating factors included the impacts of statutory over-crowding when relatives and family requested support and began to co-reside in often poor quality accommodation and debt occurring as a result of low-income employment or reliance on benefits for families which were typically bigger than majority White families. Unemployment among BME families (particularly Bangladeshi, Black Caribbean males and Pakistanis) was found – and still continues to be – greatly in excess of that among White British populations significantly increasing the risk of depression, anxiety, malnutrition and poverty-related homelessness.

Discrimination and hate crimes against some BME families (those individuals who are isolated from their community, living in rural areas or where they are relatively conspicuous may be particularly vulnerable) may also lead to homelessness applications or 'hidden homelessness', where households abandon their homes to escape discrimination (see further McDonald 2009 for a discussion on racist hate crime in Belfast).

Although national level research into the rate at which BME households become homeless or insecurely housed is somewhat outdated, the relatively rapid growth rate of some BME populations, sensitivity of particular BME populations working in insecure or casual employment to work loss and changing demographics fuelled by migration patterns (including East European migration: see further Chapter 12) means that BME populations are at particular and increasing risk of experiencing homelessness or of remaining 'hidden' and unable to access appropriate services. Phillips (2008) notes that while a growth in demand for affordable homes is found among all minority ethnic groups, the greatest need is experienced among British Pakistani and Bangladeshi families, because of their youthful age structure, early rates of marriage and new household formation and high rates of overcrowding in parental homes. An extremely high number of young people from these communities are particularly vulnerable to accommodation pressure because of their weak position in the employment market which exacerbates difficulties in obtaining decent housing in their preferred localities where existing support systems are in place.

Disability

The available literature on disability among homeless and insecurely accom-modated people tends to focus on mental health needs (see above). As explored elsewhere in this chapter, anxiety, depression and 'major' mental health needs are extremely common among people experiencing all kinds of housing crisis. In contrast, very little literature exists in relation to physical and learning disa-bility among homeless people although anecdotally, significant impairments and disabilities associated with accidents and substance use (e.g. loss of mobility or amputations following drug-related infections and abscesses) are common among street homeless, particularly those people who are sleeping rough or who have a long history of alcohol use (see e.g. interviewees profiled in Peck 2008). Doherty (2006) reports that homeless disabled people are (at least in Scotland) more likely to be accepted by local authorities as in need of priority housing and should therefore (in theory) be able to access appropriate support services at an early stage. In practice, however, the shortage of suitably adapted accommodation particularly for wheelchair users has created a significant backlog with many disabled people being forced to remain in short-term hostel accommodation while awaiting rehousing. Not only are facilities in some hostels not best suited for individuals with particular types of disability – for example those who are learning disabled or have sensory impairment – but the risk factors detailed above, particularly those related to other service users, may expose already vulnerable individuals to harm or risk of exploitation.

Peck (2008), discussing the prioritization of disabled people in homeless-ness strategies, acknowledges that the structural barriers to be faced in accessing accommodation (e.g. offers of unsuitable temporary accommodation where a resident might experience bullying in relation to their health condition or early loss of tenancy related to difficulties in adjustment to housing) can lead to a 'revolving door' cycle where even the most extremely physically disabled people return to living on the streets. Sin et al. (2009), in their review of disa-bled people's experiences of hate crime, note that physically disabled homeless or those accessing hostels can be particularly vulnerable to abuse or violence. Individuals with mental health problems or learning disabilities, while likely to be offered priority social housing at a faster rate than physically disabled homeless people, are, it should be noted, potentially at greater risk of loss of tenancy as a result of difficulties managing independent or semi-supported living, or (particularly for people with mental health issues) anti-social behav-iour. Where intersectionality occurs – for example in the call of disabled BME people – particular concerns exist that the most obvious issue (e.g. mental health or physical impairment support needs) may be prioritized, leaving an individual insufficiently supported in dealing with inequalities which exist because of other personal characteristics (e.g experiences of racism or social and cultural isolation).

Sexual orientation

Only limited research and policy notice has been taken of the role of discrimination and exclusion in relation to sexual orientation and how this increases the risk of homelessness for some people. While the Equality Act protects lesbian, gay, bi-sexual and transgender (LGBT) people from discrimination in relation to access to services (for example it would be unlawful for a gay person to be refused the opportunity to rent a flat because of their sexual orientation), anecdotal evidence suggests that young people in particular may face family breakdown, violence and rejection on 'coming out' (see further Chapter 10).

Cochran et al. (2002), in one of the few psychological studies on outcome for young homeless LGBT people in America, found that this group left home more frequently, were victims of crime more often, used more (and more addictive) substances at a greater rate of frequency than their heterosexual counterparts and had more sexual partners with whom they had an increased tendency to practise unsafe sex, sometimes in sex-work/prostitution settings. Anecdotally, young British LGBT people who are homeless or insecurely housed also report that they are at risk from other street homeless, hostel, squat or multiple occupancy housing residents who are prejudiced and heterosexist and who may behave violently towards someone on the basis of their sexual orientation.

In two studies of housing needs and social exclusion experienced by LGBT people the national charity Stonewall has reported on the considerable degree of exclusion, violence, prejudice and unthinking discrimination experienced by LGBT people across the life-course – ranging from (Stonewall Housing & Shelter 2005; Stonewall (Scotland) and the Scottish Housing Regulator 2009) rejection by family members in youth, to a marked reluctance among older LGBT people to access housing and support services as a result of their experiences in former decades when prejudice on the grounds of sexual orientation was even more common. For older or disabled LGBT people in particular, fear of how they might be treated by carers may act as a significant barrier to coming out or acknowledging their feelings towards or existing relationship with another resident of a shared house, hostel or supported housing complex.

Good practice guidance on working with LGBT homeless people (e.g Stonewall (Scotland) and the Scottish Housing Regulator 2009) stresses that for a significant minority of LGBT people harassment in the home and neighbourhood is a problem, leading some individuals to move home to avoid harassment. Barriers to engagement include the difficulties of dealing with service providers, assumptions which are exacerbated by a lack of professional awareness and training on LGBT issues. Accepting offers of accommodation (particularly in shared houses) can be problematic for some LGBT people who fear intimidation or harassment and many people – particularly women – would prefer the option of living in either female-only (preferably lesbian) or LGBT only accommodation.

Religion

Religion qua religion is rarely a specific issue in relation to homelessness and insecure accommodation in Britain. However, in many cases religious faith and belief can be regarded as a proxy for ethnicity and may, as a result of cultural practices and faith-based beliefs (e.g. in relation to use of contraception and thus family size, or attitudes to sexual orientation), impact across numerous domains. As noted earlier, Bangladeshi and Pakistani families are typically larger and more socially excluded in relation to accommodation issues and access to employment than the surrounding population. The vast majority of people from these communities follow the Islamic faith. Irish Travellers (see further Chapter 11) who also experience significant accommodation-related difficulties, are in many cases devout Roman Catholics and accordingly have a tendency to have larger families with associated impacts on over-crowding and levels of poverty.

Homelessness and insecure accommodation in relation to faith and religious belief are therefore overwhelmingly issues of inter-sectionality. Cultural and faith-based beliefs in relation to sexual orientation have been increasingly noted as causing conflict in family relations, with some LGBT charities reporting that young BME people face an even greater risk of homelessness on coming out than do their white British peers. The *Pink News* (2010) cited staff at the Albert Kennedy Trust reporting seeing clients who had been 'chased out of the house with knives and we have had issues around young people who had exorcisms planned to get rid of the gay demons' and noted that 'after young men and women in Muslim families reveal their sexual orientation, they are often asked to leave'. Other young people from BME communities report that their families have in some cases resorted to violence or imprisonment, or have arranged marriages for them to 'cure' them of being lesbian or gay (see further Hill and McVeigh 2010).

Conclusion

While homelessness may affect any individual and is often associated with a cascade of unfortunate events such as job loss or marital breakdown, certain vulnerable adults (and young people) are at greatly increased risk of experiencing insecure accommodation. Being a member of a supportive family or community network and having the ability to access finances sufficient to meet housing needs (e.g. through obtaining a deposit on a rented property) are both the main protective factors against homelessness and the routes out of such a situation in a period of declining access to public (RSL) housing.

Policy preoccupations have until relatively recently failed to take account of the complexities of homelessness and the ease with which apparently 'secure' people can become insecurely accommodated. Most models of engagement have focused on young or particularly visible 'street homeless', ignoring the plight of the 'hidden homeless' who may be of any age and experiencing significant degrees of social exclusion behind closed doors, particularly when faced with other issues, for example being a member of a minority community or having a disability. The intersectional risks which increase the likelihood of a person becoming homeless are exacerbated by lack of capitals (e.g. educational, social and cultural) which are associated with poverty and growing up in a work-poor home, or having been in an institutional setting such as psychiatric hospitals, the care system or the armed forces. In a rapidly changing postmodern world in recession, while it may be possible to predict who may experience a greater likelihood of 'falling through the net', practitioners should be alert to the risk that any client or service user may be at risk of homelessness.

Good practice in relation to working with homeless and insecurely accommodated people should involve the development of inter-agency networks of expertise and advice which can tailor support to the individual needs of a client. It is important that anyone who has contact with a homeless or potentially homeless person has familiarity with and awareness of, all domains of exclusion to ensure that responding to the most 'obvious' issue or characteristic of an individual (or family) does not exacerbate and heighten the risks they face, leading to the risk of placement failure; a cycle of deepening social exclusion and on-going homelessness or a history of short-term accommodation.

Chapter summary

- Homelessness and residence in insecure accommodation have a multi-faceted and complex impact on life opportunities, negatively impacting on all aspects of an individual's well-being.
- While some personal characteristics (e.g. age, disability, sexual orientation, ethnicity) may increase the likelihood of an individual being at risk of becoming homeless or insecure accommodated, there is no single cause or predictive factor which explains the phenomenon.
- While there is an extremely high rate of mental illness among homeless and insecurely accommodated people, this may result from earlier life

traumas or have developed as a result of the accommodation insecurity they face.

- The majority of homeless or insecurely accommodated people are 'hidden homeless' living in poor quality or over-crowded accommodation where they often have no legal right to remain.
- Education, employment and training are difficult to access and sustain when homeless.

Notes

1 For example see three cases leading to deaths reported in 2009 and 2010 in England: www.mirror.co.uk/news/top-stories/2010/05/23/homeless-man-killed-for-his-cigs-115875-22278462/; news.sky.com/skynews/Home/UK-News/Two-15-Year-Old-Boys-Charged-With-Murder-Of-Homeless-Man-In-Church-yard-In-Darlington/Article/201006415656093 and www.independent.co.uk/news/uk/crime/killing-of-a-good-samaritan-1701098.html

2 Considerable anecdotal evidence suggests that in common with insecurely sited Gypsies and Travellers (see further Chapter 11) homeless and insecurely accommodated individuals are more likely to seek help for treatable conditions at a significantly later stage of their illness than are those who have access to a secure place to live. The necessity of meeting their primary needs such as access to food or a place to sleep (identified under Maslow's (1943) hierarchy of need as a basic physiological necessity – see further Chapter 11), and the tendency to compare their health status with that of individuals in a similar complex situation, means that it is often not until their health has deteriorated until it is virtually impossible to continue with their daily routine or they are unable to ignore a chronic condition, that a homeless person will seek medical aid. In such circumstances medical professionals report that both physical and mental health has often deteriorated significantly prior to the individual being treated, leading to greater recovery times and sometimes irreparable deterioriation.

3 See for example the summary review of newspaper reported incidents of hate crimes perpetrated against disabled people in a three month period in 2010 (Novis 2010).

References

Ashmore, J. (2010) The Act. *The Pavement: The Free Magazine for Homeless people in London and Scotland*, 7 July. Available at: www.thepavement.org.uk/story.php?story=1054.

Bines, W. (1994) *Health of Single Homeless People* York: Centre for Housing Policy/ University of York.

Bowcott, O. (2009) *UK should adopt pioneering Scottish homelessness law, says UN. Guardian*, 3 June. Available at: www.guardian.co.uk/society/2009/jun/03/ un-scottish-homelessness-law-recommendations-housing.

Casey, R., Goudie, R., and Reeve, K. (2007) Resistance and identity: homeless women's use of public spaces. *People, Place & Policy Online*, 1(2): 90–7.

Centrepoint (2006) *A Place to Call Home: Care Leavers' Experience of Finding Suitable Accommodation*. London: Centrepoint. www.leavingcare.org/data/tmp/2149-4944.pdf.

Cochran, B., Stewart, A., Ginzler, J. and Cauce, A.-M. (2002) Challenges faced by homeless sexual minorities: comparison of gay, lesbian, bisexual, and trans-gender homeless adolescents with their heterosexual counterparts. *American Journal of Public Health*, 92(5): 773–7.

Communities and Local Government/ CSIP Housing Learning and Improvement Network (2008) *Understanding Homelessness and Mental Health: Housing Briefing*. London: Care Services Improvement Partnership/Housing Learning and Improvement Network; Great Britain/Department for Communities and Local Government.

Coombes, R. (2004) Falling through the cracks. *Guardian*, 13 October. Available at: http://society.guardian.co.uk/homelessness/story/0,,1325383,00.html.

Cooper, K. (2005) Court backs evictions of 'innocents'. *Inside Housing Magazine*, 6 January.

Crisis (1996) *Still Dying for a Home*. London: Crisis.

Crisis (2006) *Homeless Women: Still Being Failed yet Striving to Survive*. London: Crisis.

Crisis (2009) *Mental Ill Health in the Adult Single Homeless Population*. London: Crisis.

Dean, R. and Craig, T. (1999) *Pressure Points: Why People with Mental Health Problems Become Homeless*. London: Crisis.

Department for Social Development Northern Ireland (DSDNI) (2007) *Including the Homeless: A Strategy to Promote the Social Inclusion of Homeless People and Those at Risk of Becoming Homeless in Northern Ireland*. Belfast: DSDNI.

Doherty, K. (2006) *Housing Homeless Disabled People*. Edinburgh: Shelter (Scotland).

Frith, M. (2003) Hidden homeless at 40,000 says first survey. *Independent*, 4 November. Available at: www.independent.co.uk/news/uk/this-britain/ hidden-homeless-at-400000-says-first-survey-734500.html.

Frost, A., Corker, S., Reynolds, L. and Albanese, F. (2009) *For Whose Benefit? A Study Monitoring the Implementation of Local Housing Allowance*. London: Shelter.

Garvie, D. (2004) *The Black and Minority Ethnic Housing Crisis*. London: Shelter.

Goffman, E. (1968) *Stigma: Notes on the Management of Spoiled Identity*. London: Penguin.

Harker, L. (2006) *Chance of a Lifetime*. London: Shelter.

Health Development Agency (2004) *Homelessness, Smoking and Health*. London: HDA.

Hill, A. and McVeigh, K. (2010) Gay men become victims of forced marriages. *Guardian*, 1 July. Available at: www.guardian.co.uk/world/2010/jul/01/gay-men-forced-marriage.

Homeless Link (2009) *Survey of Needs and Provision (SNAP)*. London: Homeless Link.

Lakhani, N. and Merrick, J. (2008) 'Shocking' rise in homelessness among women *Independent*, 3 August. Available at: www.independent.co.uk/news/uk/home-news/shocking-rise-in-homelessness-among-women-883769.html.

Maslow, A. (1943) A theory of human motivation. *Psychological Review*, 50(4): 370–96.

McDonald, H. (2009) Hindu priest to flee home in Belfast after attacks. *Guardian*, 24 June. Available at: www.guardian.co.uk/uk/2009/jun/24/hindu-priest-belfast-attacks.

May, J., Johnsen, S. and Cloke, P. (2007) Alternative cartographies of homelessness: rendering visible British women's experiences of 'visible' homelessness'. *Gender, Place and Culture*, 14(2): 121–40.

Morris, M. and Easton, C. (2008) *Narrowing the Gap in Outcomes: Further Overview of Data and Evidence on the ECM Outcomes for Vulnerable Groups*. Slough: NFER.

New Policy Institute/Crisis (2004) *How Many, How Much? Single Homelessness and the Question of Numbers and Cost*. London: Crisis/New Policy Institute.

Novis, A. (2010) *Snapshot Report of Targeted Hostility towards Disabled People in the UK*. London: UKDPC.

O'Grady, S. (2010) Osborne's cap on housing benefits will 'drive poor families into ghettos'. *Independent*, 12 July. Available at: www.independent.co.uk/news/uk/politics/osbornes-cap-on-housing-benefits-will-drive-poor-families-into-ghettos-2024372.html.

Office of the Deputy Prime Minister (ODPM) (2004) *The Impact of Overcrowding on Health and Education: A Review of Evidence and Literature*. London: ODPM.

Office of the Deputy Prime Minister (ODPM) (2003) *Housing and BME Communities: Review of the Evidence Base*. London: ODPM.

Office of the Deputy Prime Minister (ODPM) (2005) *Causes of Homelessness in Ethnic Minority Communities*. London: ODPM.

Pannell, J. (2005) *Extra Care Housing Models and Older Homeless People: Housing Learning and Improvement Network. Factsheet number 16*. London: Department of Health.

Peck, S. (2008) Down on the streets. *Disability Now*, 1 April. Available at: www.disabilitynow.org.uk/living/features/down-on-the-streets.

Penny, L. (2010) The housing gap. *The New Stateman*, 15 August. Available at: www.newstatesman.com/blogs/laurie-penny/2010/08/living-young-property-house.

Phillips, D. (2008) *Black and Minority Ethnic Young People and Housing*. London: Race Equality Foundation.

Pink News (2010) Homeless charity warns of increase in gay Muslims fleeing family violence. *Pink News*, 1 November. Available at: www.pinknews.

co.uk/2010/01/11/homeless-charity-warns-of-increase-in-gay-muslims-fleeing-family-violence/.

Queens Nursing Institute (QNI) (2007) *Briefing Number 8: Health and Homelessness.* London: QNI.

Quilgars, D., Johnson, S. and Pleace, N. (2008) *Youth Homelessness in the UK.* York: Joseph Rowntree Foundation.

Ramesh, R. (2010) Homeless Poles living on barbecued rats and alcoholic handwash. *Guardian,* 12 August.

Randall, G. and Drugscope (2002) *Drug Services for Homeless People: A Good Practice Handbook.* London: ODPM.

Ravenhill, M. (2000) *Routes into Homelessness: A Study by the Centre for the Analysis of Social Exclusion of the Paths into Homelessness of Homeless Clients of the London Borough of Camden's Homeless Persons Unit.* London: Centre for the Analysis of Social Exclusion.

SECRU (2002) *Routes Out of Homelessness.* Edinburgh: SECRU.

Seenan, G. (2003) Scotland moves to end homelessness. *Guardian,* 6 March. Available at: www.guardian.co.uk/politics/2003/mar/06/housing.scotland.

Shelter (2007) *Reaching Out: A Consultation with Street Homeless People 10 Years After the Launch of the Rough Sleepers Unit.* London: Shelter.

Shelter Cymru (2010) *Living in Wales: The Housing and Homelessness Experiences of Central and East European Migrant Workers.* Cardiff: Shelter Cymru.

Sin, C.H., Hedges, A., Cook C., Mguni, N. and Comber, N. (2009) *Disabled People's Experiences of Targeted Violence and Hostility.* London: EHRC.

Smith, J. (2003) *Defining Homelessness: The Impact of Legislation on the Definition of Homelessness and on Research into Homelessness in the UK (research paper).* London: Centre for Housing and Community Research, London Metropolitan University.

Stanley, K. (2002) *Home Is Not Just a Place to Keep Our Stuff.* London: Save the Children.

Steele, A. and Ahmed, N. (2007) *Homelessness among Black Communities in the London Borough of Islington.* London: LBI/University of Salford/SHUSU/EMS.

Stein, M. (2006) Research review: young people leaving care. *Child and Family Social Work,* 11(3): 273–9.

Stonewall Housing & Shelter (2005) *Sexual Exclusion: Issues and Best Practice in Lesbian, Gay and Bisexual Housing and Homelessness.* London: Stonewall/Shelter.

Stonewall (Scotland) & The Scottish Housing Regulator (SHR) (2009) *Understanding the Housing Needs and Homelessness Experience of LGBT People in Scotland: A Guide for Social Housing Providers and Homelessness Services.* Edinburgh: Stonewall/SHR.

Williams, J. (2010) Hostel hopes to end stigma with change of name. *Sentinel Newspaper,* 22 July. Available at: http://findarticles.com/p/news-articles/sentinel-the-stoke-on-trent-uk/mi_8019/is_20100722/hostel-hopes-stigma-change/ai_n54534098/.

Wincup, E., Buckland, G. and Bayliss, R. (2003) *Youth Homelessness and Substance Abuse: Report to the Drugs and Alcohol Research Unit (a Home Office research study)*. London: Home Office Research, Development and Statistics Directorate.

Suggestions for further reading

King, P. (2003) *A Social Philosophy of Housing*. Aldershot: Ashgate.

Masters, A. (2005) *Stuart: A Life Backwards*. London: Fourth Estate.

Robinson, P. (2008) *Working with Young Homeless People*. London: Jessica Kingsley.

Seal, M. (2005) *Resettling Homeless People: Theory and Practice*. Lyme Regis: Russell House.

Taunton, M. (2009) *Fictions of the City: Class, Culture and Mass Housing in London and Paris*. Basingstoke: Palgrave Macmillan.

Tickell, J. (1997) *Turning Hopes into Homes (a History of Social Housing 1235–1996)*. London: National Housing Federation.

Wohl, A. (2001) *The Eternal Slum: Housing and Social Policy in Victorian London*. New Jersey: Transaction Publishing.

7 Substance abuse

Caroline Cole

> If you look at where so much of the burglary, so much of the car crime is coming from, it is actually coming from people who are addicted to drugs, and I think we've got to be much faster at getting drug addicts off the streets and into treatment. And all too often that doesn't happen, and even when it does today, they actually just get put on a substitute drug. And we're not really dealing with the problem which is to get these people to confront their problems and lead drug-free lives. I even went to a drug rehab recently in my own constituency and met a young man who told me that he'd committed a certain amount of crimes so he could get in front of a judge who could then get him a place in a residential rehab centre. We must be mad, as a country, not to get people into that residential rehab, get them to clean up their lives so we cut the crime on our own streets.
>
> (R. Hon. David Cameron, MP, Party Leaders' debate, April 2010)

Learning objectives

Readers of this chapter will be able to:

- describe the impact of deprivation, social exclusion and sub-cultural membership in modelling and exacerbating the potential for problematic substance use;
- challenge discourse that fails to associate 'drug use' with both legal and illegal substances (including alcohol) which cause mood alteration or (commonly) intoxication;
- contrast and where appropriate challenge the conception of substance-abuser (the demonized 'other') with the notion of a recreational-user and identify the cultural/socio-economic underpinnings of these conflicting/contrasting models;

- debate whether 'entrenched substance-related vulnerability' is inevitable, or if it is a simplistic artefact of a chaotic and inequitable system of access to treatment programmes.

Adults involved in substance abuse[1] are at risk of both suffering and perpetrating harm. Actions perpetrated under the influence of substance use often prove invidious to both self and society, and are frequently part of a pattern of wider social malaise. Vulnerability to drug use initially can be for social, emotional, psychological, genetic, economic, geographical, circumstantial or existential reasons, but once sustained drug use has taken hold, further vulnerabilities arise. When drug use has become problematic, it renders the user vulnerable to a range of health and social difficulties. Entrenched and dependent drug use is typically characterized by a chaotic lifestyle, and vulnerability to domestic violence and other forms of criminal activities may become a normative part of the user's lifestyle, in many cases leading to conviction and imprisonment.

However, despite the clear human and social cost of problematic substance misuse, interventions to support addicted individuals and to minimize harm arising from substance abuse are made deeply problematic by fragmentation and separation of various kinds. This chapter will argue that in order to effectively and holistically engage with problem substance users, three core theoretical-political approaches are required.

1. Interrogating the Drug Intervention Programme that attempts to coerce criminal justice clients into what is rhetorically termed 'effective treatment' but which fails to provide a vision for recovery and rehabilitation and thereby contributes to the 'revolving-door' phenomenon experienced by many criminal justice clients.
2. Challenging (and working with or against) sub-cultural identification which is prevalent both in the self-perceptions of problem substance users and in the differentiated responses and support networks available to them.
3. Disputing the consistent legislative position that considers that alcohol abuse should be treated in isolation from other forms of substance misuse.

The chapter will suggest that the net result of fragmented policy approaches and uncoordinated implementation of treatment options risks 'keeping people small'. While the most effective evidence-based interventions to support and rehabilitate substance-abusers are predicated upon taking a holistic approach to the issue of addiction alongside a personalized approach in working with the client,[2] the drug treatment system in Britain is riddled with inherent contradictions and inequalities of access. Service users are frequently victims of misconceptions and systemic errors inherent in treatment networks and can thus find themselves stuck in a 'revolving door cycle' of stigmatization and social exclusion which harms both themselves and others.

Keeping people outside

To some extent the language (both professional and popular) used to describe substance users – whether addicts or recreational drug users – shapes popular understanding of the issue in Britain today. The use of linguistic techniques which routinely characterize the drug user as 'outcast' and 'outsider' maintains a normative-deviant paradigm that is unhelpful in addressing both the overall issue and the vulnerabilities and problems of people who self-medicate in ways that cause harm to themselves and society.

Precisely where the line is drawn between 'insider' (an individual who is socially compliant or considered to be merely 'experimenting' with substances) and 'outsider' (the deviant 'other' cf. Cohen 1973/2002 who is invoked whenever a 'moral panic' occurs) will to some extent vary according to which substances an individual might at some stage have adopted her/himself and what drugs s/he wishes to configure as 'other', or deviant. Fuelled by the often uninformed and sensationalist media representations of drug users, the typical exclusion of alcohol from perceptions of 'drugs', and the demonstrable link between drugs and crime, such characterizations of substance-users cast some individuals 'beyond the pale', figuring them as 'folk devils' (Cohen 1973/2002) in a manner which enables us to deny the hedonism, egocentricity and savagery which is common to post-modern societies.

A number of commentators have charted this social construction of the substance-abuser as 'other'. Lenson (1995) evocatively states:

> We have drawn a circle of discourse and depiction around the lives of drug users because we would not want to relinquish our own social control to the point of ecstasy, of 'standing outside of ourselves.' And because we do not want this for ourselves, we reject all representations of it, afraid, perhaps, of some involuntary empathy.

Kohn (1997: 3) traces how historical discourse has effectively linked the otherness of drug-users to perceived otherness of racial groups by focusing on the alien nature of both the substances used and the user:

> As always, drugs are feared because of their otherness. In the late 1920s, the menace they were believed to pose found its most acute

expression in fears of miscegenation. Similar alarms were sounded in a reprise that developed after the Second World War, this time revolving round marijuana and black men instead of cocaine, opium and Chinese men. In the 1980s, the symbolism took more elliptical forms, but drugs reappeared as a means of expressing fears of a foreign threat to a nation unsure about its fortune and direction . . . At present . . . the otherness of drugs that the dominant culture seems to fear above all is not that of race, or crime, but the other world of hallucinatory states . . . As long as drugs remain illegal, so will their power to serve as symbols of deeper fears.

The 'chemical carnival' or 'rites of passage' conception of substance use

Not all individuals are presented as *dangerous* outsiders however. Those people who enjoy a certain degree of notoriety and celebrity appear to hail from the right cultural milieu, possess high degrees of social and cultural capital (Bourdieu 1986) and figure in a more complex and symbiotic relationship with the media and society at large. Press pictures of a gaunt and haunted Pete Doherty,[3] his hat askance and a cigarette hanging from his mouth suggest an artistic angst and isolation, underlined by his musical talent, reminiscent of portrayals of now canonized poets and artists of the Romantic period. Despite the averred media disapproval of the musician's lifestyle such images hold attraction for a generation obsessed with celebrity and narcissism. A different sort of outsider (more pathetic than dangerous), Doherty is particularly renowned for his heroin use, a drug that is presented in the media and popular discourse, along with crack cocaine, as responsible for most of the substance-related ills of society.

A further example (this time associated with recreational rather than addictive substance use) reveals how class and status provoke a more tolerant response in media representations. Following revelations that the young Prince Harry had been caught smoking cannabis, a newspaper article (Curtis 2002) published a feature entitled 'When Harry Met 'Arry' that identified the difference between a 'wild child' and a 'yob'. The author concludes that there is no substantive difference other than one has rich parents and, contiguous with that, is protected from both the consequences of his actions and vilification by the media. The article goes on to detail some salient differences in lifestyle that exemplify the way in which the classes are perceived, corralled and, in the case of the privileged, protected. The article is rounded off with a comment on the future prospects of the respective drug users, one as a privileged member of the royal family, the other as career criminal. Images which accompany the text present the Prince twice, once in the garb of royalty and affluence (fashionable casual trousers – belted – with check shirt and suede shoes) and the other manipulated to show him in council estate chain-store chic (combat trousers, hoodie with 'EMINEM' logo, suede trainers). The postures and physiognomy are different also, with Harry casually posed and sporting a smile, and the socially excluded/displaced 'Arry wearing a more aggressive facial expression and offering a hip-hop gesture with arms and hands. The visual representations are backed up by social and linguistic differentials between the two beginning:

> Normally the headline 'Estate boy smokes joint, has drink' would not cause the newspaper-reading public to turn a hair. This weekend, though, the estate concerned was of the country rather than the council variety, the 17-year old boy concerned was (and is) third in line to the throne, and the Royal Family found itself having another bad heir day. The responses to Prince Harry's underage boozing and illegal spliff-toking at Highgrove proved that the double standards of the class system are alive and well. While the prince's antics provoked shock, sympathy and pages of debate, similar behaviour by a 17-year old boy from a one-parent family on a sink estate would surely be seen as typical underclass yobbery.

From these two high-profile examples it is clear that the normative-deviant paradigm is not the only model available for considering substance abuse. Doherty and Prince Harry are treated in these examples in a manner which suggests that youthful excess and/or social indulgence in drugs might ultimately represent a phase or rite of passage, from which the individual will yet emerge as a responsible member of society.[4] The concept of a 'chemical carnival' (Van Ree 1997; South 1999) is an evocative and useful phrase for contemplating models of drug use. Since medieval times, the term 'carnival' has traditionally signalled a temporary upending of society and collective values that are subsequently brought back into order by the power of social organization and ritual, most clearly illustrated by the carnival before lent (Bakhtin 2009). The principle behind a contained and legitimized expression of 'otherness', permitted (at least unofficially) by the powers that be and then brought back into sobriety and conformity, is that such periods of temporary controlled wildness prevents any radical and revolutionary action that would threaten the *status quo* and the stability of the dominant society. It also sets the framework for what is acceptable and respectable by enabling people to move outside of society temporarily and parodically in order to return all the more emphatically to settled order at the carnival's end (e.g. young people ending university and entering the world of work are expected to be more 'sober' – in a number of senses – than when they are students). Although post-modern western cultures have largely lost awareness of the transient and controlled wildness associated with 'carnival', the notion of a period when many young people experiment with drugs (the time of chemical carnival) helps to clarify the boundaries of what is safe and within social control and order, and what is unusually dangerous and threatening. Moreover, not only does a model which impresses the transient nature of substance-misuse enable a perception that all is well with society, but it can be utilized to minimize the fear of danger and chaos which threatens the well-being of more than the individual substance user.

Unfortunately, the depiction of addicts as 'other', in contrast to a 'rites of passage' model, does not promise return to the fold that the carnival implies, nor is the venture into addiction parodic and harmless as is the pseudo-anti-social behaviour of the carnival participants. The addict remains an outsider unless she or he undergoes rehabilitation and reform over a long enough period to be re-assumed into mainstream society.

The carnival parallel is thus inexact but it does capture something of the inequality reflected by the press story considered earlier. Far from there being a strict line in the sand beyond which there is no return, the cases of the two protagonists suggest there is a degree of societal indulgence for a certain category of youth to engage in the 'chemical carnival', almost as a required rite of passage, the firm expectation being that this period of carnival or riotous youth will be for a fixed time only and then the libertine will ultimately rejoin society as a respectable individual. Moreover, an important socio-economic truth is revealed by the humorous and satirical swagger of the article: if you are middle or upper class and affluent and use drugs in a way that makes your life unmanageable, you *have* a problem. If you are working class and poor and use drugs in a way that makes your life unmanageable, you *are* a problem.

Class, capital and access to resources: configuring substance misuse

The preceding debate brings us to the main challenge in evolving coherent and effective interventions for adults who are (or may become vulnerable) through their drug use. There is strict demarcation between middle-class affluent drug users and working-class users. The latter are more likely to be studied and assisted with mandated interventions, and are often easier to identify than are their middle-class counterparts, having less to lose if they are 'found out' and identified. By contrast, middle-class users are frequently shielded from the consequences of their substance use by virtue of their being affluent enough to access private treatment, or through support from family, friends and medical professionals. The overall value of the cultural and social capitals they have at their disposal to tap into in times of need (frequently even when criminal justice engagement has occurred) prove more beneficial than the networks available to members of the working classes.

The following two hypothesized scenarios demonstrate the 'escape routes' from addiction which are available to people in distinct social milieus. In both cases the protagonists are female and in their early middle age.

Scenario for reflection 1

After years of incapacitating alcohol abuse, a street drinker resolves to seek assistance after experiencing a life-threatening event which occurred because she was highly intoxicated and placed herself in significant danger.

She has three options:

1) make herself known to social services and request a community care assessment to which she is entitled (although about which she probably has no knowledge);
2) approach her local DAAT (Drug and Alcohol Action Team) and be put to the bottom of the waiting list behind all the users of Class A drugs (i.e. heroin, crack cocaine);
3) go to her local alcohol support agency which, because of many (most) local authority commissioning decisions that favour the cheap option of brief intervention, will probably be unable to cater for her level of dependency and so will refer her on to the DAAT (and the waiting list) for an in-patient detoxification or encourage her attendance at Alcoholics Anonymous in conjunction with a request for a community detoxification from her GP (with whom, as a street drinker, she is probably not registered and who is unlikely to risk a community detoxification since she is homeless and without support).

Such is the plight and the vulnerability of the working-class (or underclass) street drinker.

Scenario for reflection 2

A barrister who lives in the Home Counties consumes a bottle of fine wine on her First Class train journey home from work, pops into the pub for a few glasses of wine when she alights from the train, warms herself with an aperitif before dinner and another half bottle while dining, and tops off her alcohol consumption with a 'small nightcap' before bed. This is a daily ritual, and while she feels perhaps she drinks a little more than may be sensible, she justifies it as her way of dealing with the stresses of her profession.

> The barrister may well be drinking more than the impoverished street drinker, and the dependence and dangers of withdrawal are equally dramatic, but in public, if noticed at all, she is likely to be deemed a respectable 'heavy drinker' while the other is seen as a 'hopeless alcoholic'.
>
> If and when the middle-class drinker admits defeat (or is forced to do so by those close enough to see the consequences of the drinking), she would be admitted to an expensive (and in most cases, effective) private treatment centre which would be paid for by her private medical insurance. She would receive a medically supervised in-patient detoxification and be treated psychosocially for the addiction for as long as is necessary to ensure an alliance is formed with the 12-step fellowship of Alcoholics Anonymous, and the likelihood of relapse reduced to a minimum.

As we shall see, the distinction both in *perceptions* of substance use and users and in the resources available to them, implicitly informs our fragmented approach to the rehabilitation of drug users, there being a differential system of treatment dependent upon the economic and class status of the individual seeking intervention for her/his substance use.[5]

Since the most impoverished and dependent substance users are often criminal justice clients (and not infrequently members of black and minority ethnic communities or other vulnerable groups; see further United Kingdom Drugs Policy Commission (UKDPC) 2008) and because the government considers them to be high priority for treatment in order to reduce crime, individuals convicted of criminal offences are fast-tracked into treatment. However, not necessarily, and in fact, not usually, are they referred to a treatment that works. Publicly available resources are often of variable quality and may not be effective (UKPDC 2008). Although they may jump the queue, they still nevertheless tend to be deprived of the kind of treatment available to those who can afford to pay. In any event, clear lines of causation exist between deprivation, fragmentation of social bonds, poverty and cycles of relapse even for those who have accessed substance misuse treatment (Shaw et al. 2007).

Disjointed and fragmented understanding characterizes the implementation of drug policies and it becomes difficult to evolve a discourse and interventions strategy that recognizes the degree of nuance required to devise effective interventions and cater for substance misusers in a fair and equitable way. For interventions to be effective in the long term, there must be recourse to a coordinated and holistic approach to working with substance users, an understanding of different kinds of drug use with a resulting need for different approaches, a recognition of the complexity, diversity and associated needs of problematic drug users themselves – and effective treatment regimes built upon this knowledge.

Keeping people apart

A further form of separation challenging those who work with vulnerable substance abusers is the emergence of differing subcultures which effectively keep people apart. Drug users are 'ghettoized' by public perceptions of their otherness, by the language used about them and by the surrounding architecture, culture and conditions in which addiction is fostered. This context of social displacement can reinforce identification with otherness, nihilism and addictive behaviours (Thomas et al. 2008).

Mark's tale (Stacey 2002) affords a clear example of this phenomenon, illustrating the geographical and cultural context and surrounding influences that can help to isolate an individual and shape their prospects. In this narrative, the protagonist (Mark) grew up on the White City estate in West London which is notorious for its poverty and high levels of deprivation. His schooling is typical of many people who eventually end up in prison:

> I started bunking off and hanging around with other kids who were out of school. Nobody cared about us and we didn't care about anybody else, I first smoked dope then; I was just 14 . . . At 15 I did my first burglary . . . getting the drugs was easy, everything was available on the White City Estate. (2002: 21)

The geography of exclusion typically represented by marginalized spaces such as roadside or neglected local authority-provided Gypsy and Traveller sites (see Chapters 6 and 11), high-rise flats and prison landings, all contribute to 'ghettoization'[6] via the combination of systemic neglect coupled with an often brutalized form of architecture that seeps into the psyche and manifests as despair and rage. Characterized by poverty, deprivation, hopelessness and accompanying criminality, such locales become no-go areas in which inhabitants are isolated, often even from one another, segregated from the rest of society and its benefits, and seen by mainstream culture as sites of fear and terror. It is no wonder, then, that people such as 'Mark' (Stacey 2002) find themselves in prison, in a setting which may feel oddly familiar for an individual who has experienced little agency in their life or opportunity to move beyond the bounded horizons of their locale.

Self-exclusion or inclusive 'alternative' worlds?

Both ghettoized localities and other forms of closed societies share certain characteristic markers which mark out the 'insider' and the 'outsider' – creating an ability to recognize someone who 'belongs' to a particular setting, or who can 'pass' (Goffman 1968) in a situation where to be 'other' would lead to stigmatization. For substance users, identifying markers may be the use of specific linguistic patterns and slang words, or for gang members, a particular way of dressing or specialist knowledge of an area.

Prisons are especially prone to retain the mystique of 'otherness', due to their impenetrability not only in terms of physical environment, but also in terms of sub-culture. The language of prisons, with the acronym-ridden occupational dialect of the officers, and the constant tendency of prisoners to reinvent the lexicon in order to remain unintelligible to the authority that confines them, reinforces separation and creates a mythologized (and demonized) place of otherness. This sense of exclusion and self-enforced community (where only those who have experienced the environment can understand or communicate), along with the walls that both confine and exclude, maintains the ghettoization of prisoners.

By definition, the underclass status of prisoners is reinforced in prison and yet, ironically (and traditionally when considering the historical origins of ghettos where marginalized minority communities – particularly Jews – have been confined by hostile authorities) ghettoes are where the marginalized learn to resist, challenge and undermine authority – minimizing the capacity of individuals to transcend a cycle of criminalization, substance misuse and poverty of opportunity.

Separation (and ghettoization), whether inside or outside of prison settings, may be adopted and reinforced by drug users themselves as affording the only marker of identity available to them in their marginalized *habitus* and in the absence of access to other capitals and resources (Bourdieu 1986). Ironically, the secrecy and mystique of prison allow the media its fanciful depictions of prisons as 'holiday camps' and the like. The semiotics of proficiency within the prison system, for example such as home-made tattoos, especially facial ones, mark the wearer as competent in prison culture, thereby protecting him[7] from violence and bullying. They signal his 'belonging' in this specialized environment. Outside the prison, however, such markers serve a different and opposing function, signifying his offender status and marginalizing him as 'other' and vulnerable in a society based upon achievement, education, relative affluence and values at odds with those assumed to be the values of offenders. They serve effectively as the mark of Cain.[8]

Once labelled with this identity, a person finds it increasingly difficult to break out of the cycle of addiction, crime and prison. In the absence of alternatives the sense of belonging offered by sub-cultures becomes ever more attractive. If marginalized individuals (e.g. gang members) have never been shown alternatives and ways of 'achieving' other than through gang culture or crime, their chances of autonomous change remain minimal. Even when released from prison, the circumstances to which many marginalized people return do not make for good preparation for a healthy and crime-free lifestyle.

Example

The 'Ghetto Boys' gang (tellingly named in recognition of the geographical, economic and cultural origins of the gang members, characterized by poverty and social exclusion and offering few opportunities to the inhabitants for escape through social mobility) from New Cross and Deptford are traditionally at odds with gangs from Charlton and Catford. The prospect of gang membership, as opposed to experiences of discrimination and exclusion in the 'wider' world, becomes increasingly attractive as youths grow into adulthood and achieve additional status in their locale as a result of their criminal and prison experiences which are regarded with disdain in external settings.

On an internet discussion board on gang culture, containing largely condemnatory postings, one commentator remarks: 'Those that don't understand these youths and the life they live shouldn't judge them. As a former member of the Peckham Boys, I'll say the society turned us all into what we are. These boys with no proper role models, no skills and little education have only known the streets and its ways, so until another way of life is orientated into them, the whole community should brace itself for further criminal activities' (Ugokwe 2009).

Thus separation, which in some settings such as prison can be imposed by outsiders, may, ironically, be internalized and self-perpetuated by individuals who are described as vulnerable. If people come to see themselves as vulnerable it can have the same effect as a disability label or a diagnosis (labels that have a complex and symbiotic relationship with vulnerability); the recipient can embrace the designation as a fixed immutable sign that prohibits change and transcendence.

Keeping people small?

While the differentials and associations discussed earlier serve to underline the social exclusion of the drug user, what popular discourse fails to consider is that the 'outcasts' of society, the perpetrators of crimes who become prisoners (and those who are typically the last people to respond to media articles or to have their voices heard) are usually victims also, vulnerable to the vagaries of their cultural circumstances and conditioning. By failing to provide the conceptual tools to empower individuals to nurture aspirations and build agency in their own treatment, it is inevitable that people seeking treatment (and service provision) are 'kept small' – perhaps too small to make changes other than on a piecemeal basis.

It follows that a crucial aspect of successful drug treatment is that of matching response, or treatment modality, to the level of need and individual circumstances and locating such responses within a broader socio-political context that takes a holistic, comprehensive, ambitious and inclusive view of recovery and rehabilitation.[9]

Understanding models of addiction

To enable practitioners to consider the challenges inherent in providing substance use interventions that are holistic enough to represent 'joined-up thinking' yet differentiated enough to take account of the nuanced and varied picture of contemporary substance abuse, it is necessary to consider the two dominant models of conceptualizing and understanding drug addiction that have informed so much contemporary policy and practice and have contributed to divisiveness and polarization within the field of drug treatment.

There are many 'models' of addiction that have emerged from studies of addicts, as distinct from recreational drug users in efforts to identify the conditions in which addiction is fostered and find solutions to the problem.[10]

Theories of addiction

Theories of addiction fall into two main categories:

- the belief in a *genetic predisposition* on the part of some individuals to substance abuse characterized by loss of control over mood altering substances. This is the predominant mode of viewing and treating addiction in the USA. See further HBO USA Today/Gallup (2006) poll which identified that the abstinence model is regarded as the most effective means of treatment for substance misuse;
- the *social model*, which attributes the addiction to a response to social conditions or experiences that enables the person to cope with pain, discomfort or trauma, and the beliefs associated with them.

Based on best available evidence it is currently impossible to formulate an unequivocal theory of addiction, other than to state that different individuals will match different models, or combinations of models. This is seen in 'self-help fellowships' where addicted people come from a wide variety of backgrounds and experiences, and are united sometimes by little more than their vulnerability to drug use and its attendant maladies. It is the experience of addiction and the way in which the individual perceives her/himself that is the universal inclusive aspect of fellowship membership, not the actual genetic, social, economic, experiential or philosophical background of the members.

Certain corollaries follow in relation to these models of addiction. Adherence to a pathological model of addiction places the addict as someone who 'suffers' from the disease and cannot control her/his drug use. They then tend to behave in a self-destructive and anti-social way to secure and protect their supply, regardless of whether that supply is legally available (as in the case of alcohol). Rejection of the idea of a genetic predisposition to addiction and adherence to a social model inevitably identifies substance misuse (rather than experimental or recreational use) as a logical escape from an intolerable reality, and continued drug use to be a way of 'managing' that pain.

Whichever lens we look through, once substance misuse is out of control, the reason behind the initial drive becomes irrelevant and subsumed in the overpowering compulsion to use drugs, whatever the cost. Thus the most effective interventions concentrate and build on the client's resilience, strengths and strategies for living without drugs, rather than conjecturing the cause of their habitual use.

Holistic interventions: the challenges for commissioners, providers and practitioners

Aligning legislative policy with practice

Historically, UK government drug strategy has been designed primarily to reduce drug-related crime through directing addicted people to treatment and fulfilling strategic targets of 'protecting neighbourhoods and families'. Currently, vehicles for local implementation consist predominantly of the following actors:

- Primary Care Trusts;
- Local Authority Drug Action Teams (DATs);
- Local Authority Drug and Alcohol Action Teams (DAATs);
- Criminal Justice Intervention Teams (CJITs) implementing the Drug Intervention Programmes (DIPs).

Cost-benefit analyses estimate that for every £1 spent on treatment, at least £9.50 is saved in crime and health costs (Godfrey et al. 2004). Much drug treatment research focuses on calculating the cost (financial) of drug use and on counting 'numbers in treatment' rather than the more challenging but more useful qualitative research that attempts to identify what works and for whom and when. Such a narrow conception may measure numbers accessing services

but fails to identify the fact that many participants are unable to access rehabilitation which is effective enough to stop their substance use or end the cycle
of drug related crime. In contrast, the study by Martin and Player (2000) focuses
on outcomes and demonstrates the effectiveness of the RAPt substance misuse
treatment programme delivered in UK prisons, backed up by a recent study
(www.rapt.org.uk) using data from the Police National Computer (PNC) that
reinforces these findings and identifies a significant reduction in reoffending
by clients who have undergone the programme.

The holistic practitioner faces similar challenges in applying conceptual
frameworks and legislative terminology to the realities of her/his everyday
practice. In successive government drug strategies, the term 'problematic drug
user' (PDU) has evolved to describe:

> a person who experiences social, psychological, physical or legal
> problems related to intoxication and/or regular excessive consump-
> tion and/or dependence as a consequence of his own use of drugs or
> other chemical substances (excluding alcohol and tobacco). (Advisory
> Council for the Misuse of Drugs 1982)

A major challenge occurs here in recognizing the dangers of alcohol which is
separated from other drugs in this definition. It can be argued that such a division is artificial and untenable in light of evidence about alcohol abuse,
excluding, as it does, a huge number of people who both suffer from addiction
and commit crime.[11] A reiteration of the distinction between alcohol and other
drugs in policy terms is found in the 2008 government drug strategy which
also narrows the definition of PDUs:

> Problem drug users (PDUs) are defined as those using opiates (eg.
> heroin, morphine, codeine) and/or crack cocaine. PDUs are of partic-
> ular interest because it is estimated they account for 99 per cent of the
> costs to society of Class A drug misuse. (Home Office 2008: 50)

Again this excludes alcohol users from classification as 'problematic drug users'
and, contiguously, from treatment opportunities, despite the fact that alcohol
is instrumental in many violent offences committed in Britain. Government
policy documents produced by administrations of both main parties
(Home Office, 1995, 1998, 2008) consolidate the division between alcohol
and other substances, emphasizing the link between drug use, anti-social
behaviour and offending at the expense of drawing parallels with heavy
alcohol use. Indeed as the high numbers of drugs users in prison testify to a
causal link between drug use and crime, the inter-relationship is far more
complex than purported by popular media and political discourse. It is only
with the new strategies of 2010–11 that this imbalance between alcohol and

other drugs is being addressed, alongside a new emphasis on all other drugs, not just Class As.

Coercion

The explicit policy link between drugs and crime has enabled the Criminal Justice Act of 1991 to implement coercive substance rehabilitation measures for offenders committing a 'trigger offence'[12] who tested positive on arrest for opiates or cocaine. As a result, Problem Drugs Users (PDUs) have been fed into 'treatment' in increasing numbers in an effort to reduce addiction and ultimately, recidivism.

The existence of these coercive measures further fractures treatment provision in Britain, creating a preferential system for offenders that can be seen to 'reward' their anti-social behaviour. In contrast, non-criminal drug users who are seeking treatment may have to wait to access services and may face the hurdles experienced by the homeless substance abuser described in example 1 (above). Indeed, it has been argued that such 'privileged' treatment of addicts involved in the criminal justice system prompts resentment and, in some cases, an inducement to commit crime. In a study on the effect of waiting for treatment, Donmall and Millar (2010: 76) report:

> There was clear resentment at arrest-referred clients being 'fast-tracked' into treatment; indeed a small number indicated that they knew people who had behaved so as to be arrested in order to secure faster access to treatment, and one interviewee had actually considered trying this: 'you need to get into trouble with the police and then they'll let you in'.

Alongside statutory (coercive) provision of treatment a raft of private treatment centres (mostly charities) exist for substance-abusing individuals offering a range of services across all tiers but requiring direct funding for individual patients. Where clients are unable to pay for their own treatment, they are entitled to a community care assessment with a social worker to ascertain whether their treatment may be funded by the local authority. Significantly, few people outside the treatment system are aware of this facility and are therefore excluded by their lack of knowledge and advice networks. In addition to these statutory and non-statutory treatment options there exist mutual aid groups, anonymous fellowships (e.g. alcoholics anonymous, narcotics anonymous, cocaine anonymous etc.) that are predicated on the therapeutic value of one addict helping another to recovery.

Delivery of services within this complex matrix of agencies is a complicated and often vexed issue, with some third-sector voluntary providers being responsible to several stakeholders that might include central government via the Ministry of Justice, the Home Office, the National Offender Management System, the National Treatment Agency and the NHS, and at a more local level, Primary Care Trusts, Local Authorities, Crime & Disorder Reduction Partnerships and Drug and Alcohol Action Teams. The sometimes conflicting requirements of these agencies can severely inhibit delivery of services to the client at the centre of this matrix. The interests and involvement of all the stakeholders, each with different agendas, often coincide into a crescendo of demands, all of which are high priority and often contradictory and through which managers and practitioners have to navigate a route that enables them to authentically support their clients.

Maintaining integrity

The National Offender Management Service strategy for 2008–11 sets the intention of

> providing drug treatment matched to individual need appropriate to individuals at the time that they are in the care of NOMS – making sure that the right people get the right intervention at the right time. This will allow practitioners to provide treatment modalities according to need, including substitution therapy or abstinence-based methods. (Ministry of Justice 2008: 18)

While this laudable aim appears reasonable, in light of the constraints common in the criminal justice system, such personalized treatment is unavailable, particularly for prisoners in custody where not all modalities are available in all prisons and clinical substance misuse teams are so short-staffed they only have to dispense medication, therefore discussion with prisoners of the benefits or problems associated with methadone dependency is compromised.[13] The much championed Integrated Drug Treatment System (IDTS), designed to 'stabilize' opiate-dependent prisoners on substitute drugs (mostly methadone) until they are able to make rational choices, has become for many a 'methadonia' where clients who want to detoxify from their methadone are unable to do so because they cannot get an appointment with a doctor to reduce dosage and move towards rehabilitation. Substitute methadone prescribing might look good on paper, and it has a place in drug treatment provision, but in practice the shortcomings and wrongful implementation make it a highway to hopelessness, a point pungently noted by Doward (2009) whose headline leads 'Methadone Makes Addicts of Prisoners'. Methadone maintenance becomes a metaphorical ghetto from which escape becomes increasingly difficult and where dependency is consolidated.[14] Thus it is particularly ironic that as recently as 2008 (Home Office 2008) the drug strategy stressed the need to ensure that addicted individuals are supported to detoxify and return to employment. The 2008 drug strategy document, *Drugs: Protecting Families and Communities* makes the bold assertion: 'we do not think it is right for the taxpayer to help sustain drug habits when individuals could be getting treatment to overcome barriers to employment'. Yet taxpayers are doing just that: paying for individuals to remain addicted to drugs via the methadone maintenance programmes in both prisons and communities.

As highlighted by the United Kingdom Drugs Policy Report (2008) the failure of many criminal justice drugs rehabilitation initiatives indicate that despite a large amount of investment in interventions for offending problematic drug users, little is known about effective sustainable treatment. Perhaps more importantly, as noted by Reuter and Stevens (2007) 'the UK invests very little in independent evaluation of the impact of drug policies' and deprives commissioners and providers of an appropriate knowledge base at great cost while permitting on-going investment in programmes of little value. Indeed, no evaluation has been undertaken of cognitive behavioural therapy programmes such as the Short Duration Programme (SDP) and Prisons Addressing Substance Related Offending (P-ASRO), initiatives which have been rolled out almost universally throughout the prison estate in the UK at significant expense. The previous government's strategic action plans included system change pilots (which were rushed in conception and implementation and were, therefore, ineffective in practice), guidance for families, and drug-free wings in prisons. These latter two objectives are just now coming into being, although similarly the research and needs analysis that would provide crucial information for commissioning is sadly absent.

Thus a central challenge for commissioners, both within the prison system and in community settings, lies in commissioning services that form part of a holistic and integrated system and that are selected according to whether the new service fits the system and contributes to a recovery-oriented agenda. All too often the professional practice of commissioners reflects a fragmented 'shopping basket' approach, where options which are not fully integrated or which leave clients partially treated and unsupported are selected, based upon half-understood reports of insufficiently evaluated 'cutting-edge' models, constructed from fragmented and sometimes partisan 'evidence'. Practitioners therefore have an important role in feeding back to managers and commissioners inherent flaws and contradictions in both particular models and the way in which drug strategies are being implemented, enabling the development of creative partnerships and ways of working which effectively serve individuals in the criminal justice system who wish to become drug free.

Reflection on practice

John is a first-time prisoner received in a busy local prison as a result of a violent offence (GBH) committed while under the influence of cocaine and alcohol. He tested positive for opiates and cocaine on arrest and was seen by an arrest referral worker in the police custody suite before being sent to court and immediately into prison on remand.

The arrest referral worker has forwarded his substance misuse assessment to the prison. The assessment identifies John as an opiate, crack and alcohol user for the past 15 years. John is seen by the clinical substance misuse team on admission and is prescribed methadone for his opiate withdrawals (having been able to prove that he is on a maintenance prescription in the community) and an alcohol detoxification after self-reporting as an alcoholic. He has been closely monitored since, and although heroin and crack withdrawals (painful and distressing as they may be) are not potentially fatal, alcohol withdrawals may be.

You are a member of the Counselling, Assessment, Referral, Advice and Throughcare (CARAT) team and, having received all the paperwork from the substance misuse team, are seeing him the morning after his reception.

John states that he wishes to remain on methadone since he feels unable to cope with life without drugs. He does, however, want to stop drinking as he is aware that this has a detrimental effect on his health and it makes him violent, to the extent that he has previously beaten up his partner in front of his six-year-old daughter.

The local prison where John is placed offers 'brief interventions', harm-minimization group-work and a range of referral options provided by the CARAT team.

A short-duration programme (SDP) designed to raise prisoners' awareness of the nature and extent of their drug use is available but there is no provision for ongoing alcohol treatment (although CARAT workers will often signpost clients to support services for when they return to the community).

As a practitioner involved with the case at this stage, what would you recommend in relation to the following issues?

- The level of dependency of the client and the length of time he has been using at this level.
- The level of motivation for change of this client.
- Other support services that may need to be involved with this client (in prison and/or in the community regardless of whether he received a custodial sentence or not).

Consider what risks John may be vulnerable to when he returns to the community.

Seizing the moment: recognizing opportunity and motivation

As the 'Reflection on Practice' above demonstrates, motivation for change and recovery does not always accompany clients who are suffering the conse- quences of their addiction. Practitioners may therefore wonder whether John would actually benefit from drug treatment since he asserts that he wishes to keep on using methadone. In such cases service users may choose to comply with interventions ostensibly to address their problems but in reality only in order to progress through the courts with helpful reports which maximize the potential for a non-custodial sentence. Nevertheless, despite John's reluctance to give up his methadone prescription, a skilled and knowledgeable practitioner would implement robust motivational techniques to encourage him to take the opportunity for change and engage in detoxification and treatment since this can sometimes produce felicitous results.

As noted earlier, coercive substance misuse treatment for criminal justice clients can be divisive and can sometimes privilege the offender over others seeking treatment, but there is more to be said of this. Initially, coercive measures were looked upon with scepticism and disapproval by some professionals in the field; scepticism about the ability of an extrinsic motiva- tion to have any real and sustainable effect on a person's behaviour, and disapproval because of a perceived compromise to the offender's rights and confidentiality. However, coercive treatment via the criminal justice system has now become a norm of treatment and research has shown – and most practitioners in rehabilitation acknowledge – that success is predicated less on the motivation with which service users enter treatment than by the motivation acquired during treatment.

In short, whether someone is in the criminal justice system or not, motiva- tion can vary on a whim and to catch and capitalize on the desire for treatment can ensure, or not, engagement and the nourishment of that motivation. Regardless of the reasons why an individual enters treatment, the most effective way of working with substance misusers is to seize the moment and build upon the desire for change. Today a client may want an unlimited supply of drugs (methadone maintenance or illegally procured drugs), tomorrow they may want to be drug free. Oscillation between these two poles is normal for a using addict, as is fluctuating preferences between treatment options and ambivalence about treatment goals. Thus flexibility and the utilization of every opportunity to engage with motivation are important tools in supporting people into recovery. Skilled practitioners will coordinate and orchestrate the client's existing recovery capital and their goals with the treatment options available as well as a vision of recovery that will support the client to aspire to greater freedom.

The following case study, written as a third-person narrative by the anonymous client herself, demonstrates this *'agency effect'* that coincides serendipitously with the internal mechanisms of the client's psyche and the impact of peers who went before to enhance motivation and provide a felicitous outcome.

CASE STUDY: EDITH

Edith had been using for 20 years and had considered herself addicted for 14 years. She was dealing in heroin to meet her own needs and as a result of a regular clientele was able to access a plentiful supply of her drug of choice.

She had previously attempted residential detoxification and had failed on more than one occasion to achieve abstinence. She considered that her own use of heroin (despite her access to a plentiful supply) was untenable and decided to enter residential treatment as a means of achieving respite. Previously, when she had attempted detoxification, Edith had left hospital still using methadone and returned to heroin use, using methadone as a back-up for when she was unable to 'score'.

On deciding to enter into residential detoxification on the last occasion Edith reported that she regarded this choice as providing a 'haven' from the daily difficulties of securing drugs and risking arrest and imprisonment but that she had lost hope of ever being able to stop using drugs. While she desired to be substance-free, she had no belief in her ability to change and regarded her 'respite' as a means of delaying the inevitable consequences of her lifestyle.

Edith's detoxification took place many years before the NICE (2007) guidelines on substance misuse treatment recommended alliance with 'mutual aid groups' for people undergoing treatment interventions. Nevertheless, the consultant psychiatrist at the hospital where Edith was treated insisted that every service user attend at least one Narcotics Anonymous (NA) meeting during their detoxification.

Two members of Narcotics Anonymous visited and facilitated a meeting on the ward where Edith was based. One of them had been 'clean and sober' for two years and the other for two-and-a-half years. The accounts they gave of their personal using histories and duration were similar to Edith's. By her own account, this proved to be the turning point for Edith during which she began to learn about the nature of addiction and the hopelessness of trying to control it, and began to see that abstinence and recovery might just be a possibility.

For the first time in nine years since coming out of prison Edith was able, with the encouragement, understanding and peer support of the NA members, to achieve methadone detoxification and complete abstinence from all mood-altering drugs. The idea of recovery had been inconceivable to her on admission, yet desire and motivation had been injected through this first encounter with other addicts who were abstinent and recovering and she kept going back to the weekly meetings, seduced by the freedom on offer there.

Recognizing the extent of her vulnerability to addiction, Edith went from the hospital detoxification programme to a 12-step treatment centre where she underwent intensive rehabilitation before returning to live in London where she forged a strong allegiance with Narcotics Anonymous.

Twenty-four years later Edith remains abstinent from all mood-altering chemicals (including alcohol), is the proud holder of several degrees, works for a pioneering organization, does 'service' helping other recovering addicts in NA, and enjoys all the rights and responsibilities of full citizenship.

Conclusion

Clear dangers exist that the conflation of the Criminal Justice System and drug treatment and the privileging of criminal justice clients over non-offenders creates a situation where some vulnerable individuals who are motivated to become substance free are unable to access services. An obsession with 'numbers' accessing services rather than quality of treatment, the resulting reduced budget per capita, and differential entry systems depending on finances and access to knowledge, networks and recovery capital, mean that the most marginalized people – who are often at greatest risk to and from substance use and crime – are frequently failed by the system when they seek advice and treatment. A tendency to conceptually and in policy terms separate alcohol users from users of other drugs and to place addicts in largely ineffectual short-term day programmes while they remain locked in their drug-using ghetto, inevitably leads to failure of treatment and a cycle of exclusion for many people who would benefit from holistic support. In addition, as the closure of numerous residential treatment centres throughout 2009 demonstrates, by diverting funds almost exclusively to the short-term measures described in this chapter, we are in danger of losing abstinence-based residential treatment centres that have demonstrated real value for money, not only in changing service users' lives (and in some cases saving lives), but in effecting the kind of radical change that benefits society when ex-users reintegrate fully and become working, tax-paying, pro-social citizens partaking of the rights and responsibilities of society – like Edith in the case study above.

With the advent in Britain in 2010 of a coalition government which lays claim to a vision of a 'Big Society' now is the time to rethink the existing system of substance treatment programmes and policies which keep people separate, 'small' and dependent and press for an holistic, tailored and comprehensive approach to delivering recovery, reintegration and abstinence services which realize service users' full human potential.

Points for reflection

1. Consider your own knowledge of and attitudes towards various types of 'drugs'. How and why do you classify these in terms of harm caused? What do you instinctively imagine when you consider an 'addict'? Are some types of substance 'users' or 'misusers' more dangerous than others – and what factors do you think are important and form part of your thought processes in imagining such a substance misuser (e.g. stereotypes; media reports, personal knowledge etc.)
2. How relevant do you think the preceding discussions on ghettoization and 'poverty of place' are to your understanding of the factors which impact on someone becoming a substance misuser? Do you personally feel if you lived in (a) a run-down estate or (b) a country estate that you would be more or less likely to become a substance misuser? If not, why?
3. Consider the challenges which might face a former addict with a criminal conviction – how might your service (or area of work for which you are training) best support a service user of this type in achieving abstinence and becoming rehabilitated into employment, education and training. What are the particular risks they might face in their day-to-day life?

Chapter summary

*   Significant discrepancy exists between rhetoric and reality of substance misuse programmes with many programmes being inadequately evaluated before they are commissioned.
*   Policy artificially separates alcohol misuse from that of other (illegal) substances so that alcohol services are frequently inadequately supported to provide appropriate treatment.
*   Fragmentation and separation in treatment options occur at all levels and functions of the system.
*   The inequitable emphasis on criminal justice interventions, statistics and short-term cost-effectiveness (which tends to exclude the long-term and 'human' costs of recidivism and failed treatment) adds to the criminal justice revolving-door syndrome characteristic of so many addicts' lives.
*   Systemic failures in 'the system' risk keeping drug users 'small' and dependent, not only on the drugs, but also on controlled substances such as methadone supplied by 'helping' agencies which are inextricably networked into processes which benefit pharmaceutical companies more than individual addicts.

- Commissioners working in the field of substance use should remain aware of the need to evaluate effectiveness in practice and outcomes and ensure that strategies and operational realities are brought closer together.
- Evidence-based practice should ensure use of qualitative techniques to identify what works for whom, when, and for how long, and attempt to recreate those conditions in response to individual need.
- A necessity exists for practitioners to engage with service users, researchers and the media to disseminate information on effective interventions, narratives of recovery and good practice in synthesizing supportive services, and use that collective knowledge to challenge the negative myths about drug users and campaign for the more effective interventions.

Notes

1   Within this chapter 'substance abuse/misuse' means the use of illegal drugs, or the problematic or illicit use of alcohol, prescribed medication, legal highs, over-the-counter medicines and volatile substances such as aerosols and glue. Misuse (utilizing the definition used by the Department for Children, Schools and Families 2011) is defined as substance taking 'which harms health or social functioning'. Substance misuse may be dependency (physical or psychological) or substance taking that is part of a wider spectrum of problematic or harmful behaviour. One-off or experimental substance use would not therefore be expected to fall within this definition.

2   The term 'user/abuser/misuser' is variously used to signal the ideological stance of the scrutinizing eye at any given moment (cf. Foucault 1973). Accordingly, when representing the 'client' perspective it may be pertinent to deploy the term 'drug-user'. When an agency or the legal system desires to exert some judgement or control over that user, however, the same person may be termed a 'drug abuser' or 'drug misuser' by the agent of the state/ labelling body. Within this theoretical model, terminology relating to drug use is mostly a matter of ideological perspective rather than empirical fact.

3   A British musician who has been notoriously associated with a cycle of heroin addiction/rehabilitation; arrest and imprisonment for a number of years.

4   A broad generalization that differentiates between social users and dependent users may be made in that the occasional, or social, user is made vulnerable *by* drug use, whereas the dependent person is vulnerable both *by* and *to* drug use.

5   Further complicating our understanding of drug culture is the popular perception of an opposition between dealer and victim that Kohn (1997: 2) claims 'belongs to a narrative that has much in common with the vampire genre'. Drug dealers are perceived as being more demonic than users and the

more successful they are the more demonic they are deemed. Yet, in reality, most dealers are dealing in order to feed their own habits and are as much a victim of the addiction as those they serve, despite not being recognized as vulnerable.

6 Typically the process by which an isolated and underprivileged urban area becomes ever more marginalized as residents find it harder to move out of the locality and poor reputation and reducing services impact on individuals willingness to become residents. Ultimately, 'ghettoized' localities contain only the most excluded individuals such as lone parents, workless households pensioners who have lived in the locality for a long time or (frequently marginalized) new migrants. Crime tends to be rife in such localities as statutory services and agencies often leave residents to 'self-police' their own neighbourhoods.

7 Facial tattoos are predominantly, but not exclusively, utilized by male prisoners.

8 Curiously, tattoos are currently fashionable and, therefore, common in our culture at present. However, the style and competence with which the tattoo has been applied clearly differentiates between stylish youths and former prisoners.

9 The term 'recovery' has recently been deployed ubiquitously in response to the new government's imperative to provide drug treatment that leads to ongoing recovery and reintegration. However, in many cases this does not signal a change in service provision but is merely a rhetorical appellation added to the same old services providing the same old interventions. It is, therefore, a politically ambiguous term that requires definition for each deployment. Here it is used to mean abstinence-based freedom from addiction that enables the participant to enter a process of becoming fully socially functional, including working, paying taxes, and adhering to the law.

10 For an initial overview of the very complex phenomena and hotly debated theories of addiction, see Sparknotes at http://www.sparknots.com/health/addiction/section2.rhtml which identifies some of the prevalent models, such as genetic, exposure biological, exposure conditioning and adaptive.

11 Some of the numerous references to alcohol's status as a common drug are available via the Royal College of Psychiatrists on http://www.rcpsych.ac.uk/mentalhealthinfoforall/problems/alcoholanddrugs/alcoholour favouritedrug.aspx. See also Edwards (2003). The author of this text is both a psychiatrist and member of the World Health Organization's Expert Advisory Panel.

12 For example, theft, robbery, burglary, sale of controlled drugs etc.

13 Methadone is not the only substitute-prescribing option but is the most popular one with medical professionals and tends still to be used more widely than buprenorphine or other drugs that offer relief from symptoms of withdrawal. This chapter speaks of methadone predominantly but other opioid agonists may be inferred by the reader as alternatives.

14   The debate as to whether diamorphine or methadone should be used as a maintenance alternative to street drugs still rages and the dominant voice remains with the methadone lobby to render methadone the drug of choice of prescribers despite research that suggests diamorphine is preferable to users and more efficacious in both preserving user health and in reducing illegal drug use. See, for example, Sell et al. (2001) and Metrebian et al. (2010).

References

Advisory Council for the Misuse of Drugs (1982) *Treatment and Rehabilitation*. London: Department of Health and Social Security.

Bakhtin, M. (2009) *Rabelais and His World* (trans. H. Iswolsky). Bloomington: Indiana University Press.

Bourdieu, P. (1986) The forms of capital. In J. Richardson (ed.) *Handbook for Theory and Research for the Sociology of Education*. New York: Greenwood.

Cohen, S. (1973/2002) *Folk Devils and Moral Panics*. London: Routledge.

Curtis, N. (2002) 'When Harry met 'Arry'. *The Evening Standard*, 15 January.

Department for Children, Schools and Families (2011) *Substance Misuse amongst Looked After Children*. London: Department for Children, Schools and Families.

Donmall, M. and Millar, T. (2010) The effect of waiting for treatment. In S. MacGregor (ed.) *Responding to Drug Misuse: Research and Policy Priorities in Health and Social Care*. Hove: Routledge.

Doward, J. (2009) Britain's prison system churns out thousands of prisoners addicted to methadone, according to a think-tank with close links to the Tories. *Observer*, 22 November.

Edwards, G. (2003) *Alcohol: The World's Favourite Drug*. New York: St Martin's Press.

Foucault, M. (1973) *The Birth of the Clinic: An Archaeology of Medical Perception*. London: Routledge.

Godfrey, C., Steward, D. and Gossop, M. (2004) Economic analysis of costs and consequences of the treatment of drug misuse: two year outcome data from the National Treatment Outcomes Research Study (NTORS). *Addiction*, 99(6): 697–707.

Goffman, E. (1968) *Stigma: Notes on the Management of Spoiled Identity*. Harmondsworth: Pelican.

HBO/USA Today (2006) *USA Drug Addiction online poll*. Available at: http://www.hbo.com/addiction/pdf/USATodayPoll.pdf.

Home Office (1995) *Tackling Drugs Together: A Strategy for England 1995–1998*. London: Home Office.

Home Office (1998) *Tackling Drugs to Build a Better Britain*. London: The Stationery Office.

Home Office (2008) *Drugs: Protecting Families and Communities: The 2008 Drug Strategy*. London: The Home Office.

Kohn, M. (1997) The chemical generation and its ancestors: dance crazes and drug panics across eight decades. *International Journal of Drugs Policy*, 8(3): 137–42.

Kohn, M. (2001) *Dope Girls: The Birth of the British Drug Underground*. London: Granta.

Lenson, D. (1995) *On Drugs*. Minneapolis, MN: University of Minnesota Press.

Martin, C. and Player, E. (2000) *Drug Treatment in Prison: An Evaluation of the RAPt Treatment Programme*. Winchester: Waterside Press.

Metrebian, N. et al. (2010) Supervised injectable heroin or injectable methadone versus optimised oral methadone as treatment for chronic heroin addicts in England after persistent failure in orthodox treatment (RIOTT): a randomised trial. *The Lancet*, 375(9727): 1885–95.

Ministry of Justice (2008) *The National Offender Management Service Drug Strategy 2008–2011*. London: NOMS/MoJ.

National Institute of Clinical Excellence (NICE) (2007) *Drug Misuse: Psychosocial Interventions and Opioid Detoxification*. London: NICE.

Reuter, P. and Stevens, A. (2007) *An Analysis of UK Drug Policy*. London: UK Drug Policy Commission.

Sell, L., Segar, G. and Merrill, J. (2001) Patients prescribed injectable opiates in the North West of England. *Drug and Alcohol Review*, 20: 57–66.

Shaw, A., Egan, J. and Gillespie, M. (2007) *Drugs and Poverty: A Literature Review*. Glasgow: Scottish Drug Forum.

South, Nigel (ed.) (1999) *Drugs, Culture, Controls and Everyday Life*. London: Sage.

Stacey, S. (ed.) (2002) *Tales from the Landings*. London: RAPt.

Thomas, Y., Richardson, D. and Cheung I. (eds) (2008) *Geography and Drug Addiction*. Berlin: Springer.

Ugokwe, K. (2009) Evening Standard on-line commentary (1–12–2009) in response to article 'Two teenage boys stabbed . . . it's just another day of gang warfare in Peckham'. Available at: http://www.thisislondon.co.uk/standard/article-23484519-two-teenage-boys-stabbed-its-just-another-day-of-gang-warfare-in-peckham.do.

United Kingdom Drugs Policy Commission (UKDPC) (2008) *Reducing Drug Use, Reducing Re-offending: Are Programmes for Problem Drug-using Offenders in the UK Supported by the Evidence?* London: UKDPC.

Van Ree, E. (1997) Fear of drugs. *International Journal of Drug Policy*, 8(2): 93–100.

Suggestions for further reading

Buchanan, J. (2004) *Missing Links? Problem Drug Use and Social Exclusion* (research paper) Glyndwr University: Social Inclusion Research Unit.

MacGregor, S. (ed.) (2010) *Responding to Drug Misuse: Research and Policy Priorities in Health and Social Care*. Hove: Routledge.

Social Exclusion Unit (SEU) (2002) *Reducing Re-offending by Ex-prisoners*. London: SEU.

8 The older person

Agnes Fanning

The publication of the No Secrets Guidance in 2000 and the subsequent promulgation of the National Service Framework for the Older Person (DoH 2001) were a major breakthrough for the older person, representing the first formal recognition of adult protection as a discrete area. The National Framework laid out a very clear context that all health professionals should work towards when caring for the older person, whether in the hospital or home setting. Both documents promote choice and empowerment for the older person, yet over ten years on from the No Secrets (DoH 2000) publication it is still evident that a number of undetected older adults continue to remain at risk. This chapter will explore reasons why abuse is still happening to many of our older citizens and will aim to give guidance on recognizing signs of abuse and possible solutions in dealing with abuse of the older person.

Learning objectives

Readers of this chapter will be able to:

- recognize that abuse to vulnerable older adults can take a variety of forms;
- identify and recognize warning signs of abuse;
- understand the legal implications of abuse of the vulnerable older person;
- identify the range of support that is available for this group of vulnerable older person.

By the very nature of our make-up we are intrinsically vulnerable and insecure (Turner 2006) and this condition can only exacerbate as we age. The publication in the first year of the millennium of *No Secrets* (DoH 2000) has proved greatly influential in raising awareness of the various types of abuse to which older vulnerable adults can be exposed. The report brought to prominence the potential risks to elderly people in both institutional and home care settings. In the ensuing decade, research has tended to concentrate on establishing the prevalence and nature of elder abuse; rather less attention has been given to recommendations for safeguarding older people and averting abuse. Informed by the current literature and policy context, the current chapter will explore practical ways of empowering the older vulnerable adult and affording them the skills to protect themselves when confronted with abuse. The chapter will consider the vital role of practitioners in developing resilience and coping strategies in this group of people by partnership working. Such a way of working, it is suggested, is best placed to assist the many older people who wish to remain in their own homes, protected and freed from fear of abuse.

The immediate policy context

The Safeguarding Vulnerable Groups Act (2006) and Safeguarding Vulnerable Groups Order (2007) represent the most immediate policy context for understanding vulnerability in the older person. These policy initiatives identified areas wherein children or adults may be deemed vulnerable or 'at risk'. A number of these areas are particularly relevant to the older person, for example if the older person is:

- living in residential accommodation, such as a care home;
- living in sheltered housing;
- receiving domiciliary care in their own home;
- receiving any form of healthcare;
- receiving a specified welfare service, namely the provision of support, assistance or advice by any person, the purpose of which is to develop an individual's capacity to live independently in accommodation or support their capacity to do so;
- receiving a service or participating in an activity for people who have particular needs because of their age or who have any form of disability;
- receiving direct payments from a local authority or health and social care trust in lieu of social care services; or
- requires assistance in the conduct of their own affairs.

Many of these contexts have the potential for the older person to be exposed to a variety of abusive situations yet the list is not exhaustive nor is the 'at risk' older person always a readily identifiable entity. How is the vulnerable older person to be recognized? Age-based classifications are arbitrary – increasingly so given increased life-expectancy, activity and resilience among the older population. Clearly, the fact that a person may be over 66 years of age is not sufficient reason *per se* to suggest that they may be a vulnerable adult.

Instead, vulnerability in the elderly, as often with other age groups, is better understood as contextual and situation-dependent. That is to say, the degree to which an individual may be deemed 'at risk' is contingent upon the situation at hand and the resilience of the individual in the context of that situation at any given time. Since our faculties, physical means and support networks all vary over the lifespan, instances can occur in which people are not always aware that they are indeed in a vulnerable situation. An older person may be at risk of physical abuse, financial neglect, environmental neglect, psychological abuse, sexual abuse or emotional abuse. Each one of these risks is major enough on their own, but many older people may be susceptible to more than one of these risks. Abuse often goes hand-in-hand with vulnerability, especially when directed at the older person or children. The Department of Health publication *No Secrets* (2000: 9) defined abuse as

> a violation of an individual's human and civil rights by any other person or persons. It may be physical, verbal or psychological, it may be an act of neglect or an omission to act, or it may occur when a vulnerable person is persuaded to enter into a financial or sexual transaction, to which he or she has not consented, or cannot consent. Abuse can occur in any relationship and may result in significant harm to, or exploitation of, the person subjected to it.

Abuse can often be very subtle, can take many forms, and may have been going on for a number of years. Where abuse may have been carried out by people known to the older person, questions need to be asked as to whether the perpetrators intentionally abuse their older relative, neighbour or friend or whether the abuse has been going on for so long that both abuser and abused may have habituated and 'normalized' such behaviour to the extent that they are not even consciously aware that abuse is occurring. Without effective identification and reporting of abuse, the potential exists for an escalation of the situation since as the older person becomes progressively less able to retaliate they become still more vulnerable.

Consciousness raising

In 2006 it was reported that one-third of the UK population had not heard of older abuse (Help the Aged 2006). Is this because certain actions are not seen as abuse or is it because society attributes limited value to the older person and characterizes them more readily as a problem rather than as a productive group of people who can contribute to society? Government pronouncements to the effect that the contributions and experiences of all citizens should be recognized and valued (DoH 2008) are not necessarily translating into coherent care packages for some of the most vulnerable people in our society and recent administrations have arguably placed greater emphasis on provision of support for younger people than for the elderly. The circular produced in December 2009 by the then Department for Children, Schools and Families continued a decade-long trend of prioritizing funding initiatives aimed at a range of children's services. By contrast, while the same time-frame has seen acknowledgement by the Department of Health of certain aspects of old age, initiatives (one being the National Dementia Strategy published in 2009) targeted at the support of the vulnerable older person have tended to be less high-profile and more time-constrained in scope. According to Kelly (2010) sufferers of dementia, on account of their perceived cognitive impairment, enjoy little legitimate voice in society anyway. Nevertheless, although the Department's policy documents consistently recognize that abuse of vulnerable adults has many parallels with that of child abuse (see e.g. DoH 2002), in terms of denial underestimation and final realization, political and media momentum tends to gather more readily around interventions to support 'the next generation' and therefore 'the future', rather than 'the older generation'. Prompted in part by the deficit in pension funds after the global recession, recent government initiatives to remove the retirement age ceiling show a step in the right direction in recognizing the economic productivity and wider societal contribution of the older person. Bytheway (1995) has drawn a connection between economic productivity and social visibility, noting that while vulnerable older people may well once have been economically productive ensuring a certain visibility in society, their retirement from economic productivity brings a corresponding decrease in visibility and an implicit assumption that their value in society is lessened as they move from self-determination to increasing dependence on others.

The corollary of this low visibility of the 'older generation' in political and media discourse is limited recognition of elder abuse in society. Yet the Action on Elder Abuse study carried out in 2007 claimed that abuse of the older person was very prevalent in the UK. The study found that 51 per cent of abuse typically involved a partner or a spouse, 49 per cent was typically perpetrated by another family member, 13 per cent by a care worker and 5 per cent by a close friend. The samples studied were representative of the UK population of residents of 66 years and over and who lived in their own private homes (Action on Elder Abuse 2007). A further study jointly funded by the Department of Health and Comic Relief (2007) found that between 2.6 per cent (227,000) and 4 per cent (342,000) of people had experienced some form of abuse or neglect compounding this dilemma. McCreadie et al. (2006) claim that less than 5 per cent of abused adults are known to the adult protection teams.

Chambers (1989: 1) suggests that vulnerability has two very different distinctions, internal and external:

> The external side of risks being shocks and stress to which an individual is subject; and an internal side which is defenceless, meaning a lack of means to cope without damaging loss. Loss can take many forms-becoming or being physically weaker, economically impoverished, socially dependent, humiliated or psychologically harmed.

However, as the fragility and dependencies of older people increase, their vulnerability also increases accordingly. It is this group of people who potentially could fall between two nets unless consciousness is consistently raised among health and social care practitioners and agencies. The Commission on Integration and Cohesion (2007) has made attempts to introduce cohesion into communities yet the main emphasis to date has been on the integration of people of different faiths, not necessarily taking account of the many older members of the community who may not belong to a particular faith. Efforts are being made to recognize the needs of the older people who live on their own. Yet this is a catch-22 situation because communities and professional and voluntary services need to know of these people living in isolation if any element of support can be given to them. The vulnerable elderly can too readily become the forgotten 'at risk' constituency and abuse can go unrecognized.

Identifying abuse of the elderly

The recent moves towards increased legal protection for vulnerable adults encourage open dialogue and establish channels for the reporting and identification of elder abuse. Warning signs of abuse are varied and will not always follow predictable trends but documented signs include examples of the once vocal and opinionated person becoming reticent and no longer speaking out; the development of a sudden habit such as rolling the hair, or twisting the fingers; refusal of assistance with personal hygiene. Other physiological changes need to be looked out for also, such as avoiding eating, incontinence, frequent fractures or bruising on limbs. This is not to say that all of these are invariably signs of abuse in the older person, but all are possible warning signs warranting careful consideration. The need for vigilance among practitioners is the more acute given the well-documented reticence among some groups of older people in self-reporting episodes of abuse. Many of the population currently over 66 years of age will have lived through the tail-end of the Second World War (indeed, many veterans may even have been actively involved in this conflict). These individuals may well have been exposed to many traumatic situations and dilemmas that are far from the common experience of the civilian. This in part may be one of many reasons why they do not always seek support in contexts of neglect, disadvantage or abuse. The need for vigilance and sensitivity among practitioners is thus crucial if silent sufferers of abuse are to be empowered and supported.

Scenario for reflection

What are the ways in which an older person might recognize that they are being abused and the channels in which they might safely report this abuse?

Imagine an older person in your case is reticent to declare an instance of abuse. What reasons might lie behind their reluctance to report the abuse?

Protecting the 'at risk' older person in diverse settings

As the state has progressively committed to providing greater protection from abuse for all vulnerable adults (DoH 2000), health and social care staff have a duty to promote this philosophy throughout every aspect of their care. The difficulty with this is that care of the elderly is carried out in a variety of settings and integrated approaches to safeguarding well-being are not always easy to achieve. The following list demonstrates the number of variants in providing formalized care.

- Residential accommodation is accommodation where any care or nursing is provided. It includes care homes registered and inspected by the Care Quality Commission in England, Care and Social Services Inspectorate in Wales and the Regulation and Quality Improvement Authority in Northern Ireland.
- Homes not registered with the Care Quality Commission, for example, small care homes for groups of adults who need assistance or support but who do need personal care.
- Controlled activity in domiciliary care includes individuals who have contact with vulnerable adults frequently or on an intensive basis, but who do not directly provide the care to the individual in their own home. Such individuals will include those who are mainly concerned with the administration of the domiciliary care service.
- Hospital care where nursing care is provided by either the NHS or Private Health Care Services.
- Home care where nursing care is delivered by a Community Nursing Team, regulated by Primary Care Trusts.

- Home care where social care is delivered by social services, regulated by social services or private agencies.

Additionally of course, there is the extensive amount of non-formalized care that is carried out in an individual's private home or in the home of a close relative or friend. Care carried out in these settings is not always monitored or regulated and, accordingly, research finds that a significant percentage of abuse of the older person often occurs in familiar surroundings and is carried out by someone well known to the dependent individual (O'Keefe et al. 2007). Indeed, it could be argued that this is the group of vulnerable adults who are most at risk because they are relying on their 'carer' to help them meet their activities of daily living. In many instances the dependent individual is reliant solely on one other person, often a spouse or a son or daughter. This group of dependent older people are the hardest audience to reach and the identification and reporting of instances of abuse among this population are particularly difficult. Concerned citizens harbouring suspicions that a neighbouring older person is subject to abuse often do not know where to go to report their concerns (Action on Elder Abuse 2008) and respect for the privacy of the individual family unit can also inhibit reporting. Yet just as recent policy directives on safeguarding children have increased the perception that abuse is everyone's business, so communities need to be encouraged to apply these same principles to the treatment of the older person. Recent government statements show a positive step in this direction:

> Safeguarding vulnerable adults who are at risk of harm sits at the heart of Government. Those who need safeguarding help are often elderly and frail, living on their own in the community, or without much family support in care homes; they are often people with physical or learning disabilities, and people with mental health needs at risk of suffering harm both in institutions and in the community. It is to these and to many others that Government have a duty of safeguarding.
>
> (Minister of State, Department of Health, Ministerial Statement, in Hope 2010)

Nevertheless, care in the community continues to be difficult to monitor. A study carried out by Action on Elder Abuse in 2008 aimed to map the extent of abuse among people aged 66 and older within their own homes. The study found that more than 6700 reports of abuse should have been documented, but only 99 referrals of abuse were in fact reported. This report did not take into account any other physical or psychological conditions which required assistance for people living at home. Kelly (2010) reaffirmed this with the results of her study, acknowledging that 70 per cent of older people said that they had reported the incident of abuse or sought help for it. However, when looking at dilemmas in elderly care, Gosney (2009) reported that only 30 per cent of help was sought from a health professional or a social worker. These statistics are very worrying and something must be done to enable the older person to feel empowered. Why do these people feel so powerless? Nahmiash (2000) suggests that many people feel ambivalence about taking action following an abuse, suggesting that this is often followed by feelings of negative self images, tiredness, anger, hurt and sadness. Any individual taking on these feelings of negativity will naturally become more withdrawn and will not feel comfortable sharing their thoughts and feelings with others. Once again this is compounded by the fact that they are possibly relying on their abuser to carry out their personal care, so may fear retribution. Mowlan et al. (2007) did not identify this as a reason in their qualitative study, but some of the reasons identified were that the abused person was unsure of the confidentiality policies. It could be suggested that if confidentiality was breached then fear of retaliation may impact on the vulnerable older person.

It would seem that psychological abuse is the most difficult type of abuse to deal with and yet Gosney (2009) suggests that it is probably the most common form of abuse. This is the one form of abuse when the perpetrator can use their 'power' without laying a finger on the abused person. Often the perpetrator continues using this method of abuse until the vulnerable person is worn out and gives into the demands or becomes so psychologically damaged that they are unaware of what is happening to them. Some suggest that a person's past oppressive experience, for example in a concentration camp, may become revived during an abusive situation, thus pushing them back into a process of powerlessness (Pritchard 2000).

Abuse within the hospital or residential setting is easier to monitor as there are health and safety policies that must be adhered to when caring for all patients or residents, not only those that are seen as 'vulnerable'. Nevertheless areas of severe neglect are still evident and have captured sporadic media attention. The Mid Staffordshire NHS Trust enquiry which reported in 2009 resulted in such headlines as the following: 'Hospital patients were left "sobbing and humiliated" by uncaring staff' (BBC News Channel, 24 February 2010). And 'Older people and their families tell us that frequently people are not getting the proper support to eat and the food is not attractive enough and as a consequence of that people are not getting a balanced diet they need and that is having a negative impact on their health' (BBC News Channel, 24 February 2010).

These examples are the more concerning given the oft-cited 'demographic timebomb' awaiting modern Britain. By 2025 the number of resident citizens 85 years old and over will increase by two-thirds, placing considerable further demand on health and social care services which, on the evidence of the mid-Staffordshire inquiry, are already strained. Reed et al. (2004) suggest that currently older people are seen by some professionals as obstacles to the fulfilment of short- and medium-term targets and as they require complex and long-term responses and interventions. With advances in medication regimes and preventative healthcare boosting life-expectancies and enabling people to live longer with long-term conditions, these challenges will only be exacerbated in the years to come.

Currently some residents in care homes have been given 'comment cards' whereby they are encouraged to alert the inspectorate to any upsetting or abusive practices (Sumner 2002). This is one method of acquiring information about abusive acts occurring. However, it may not be a very reliable system. It is possible that an older person may feel intimidated by this suggestion and may not feel comfortable about reporting an abuse. They may also feel that there could be some retaliation if the 'care' they are receiving is questioned. The Department of Health White Paper, *Our Health, Our Care, Our Say* (2006) is promoting patient choice, thus empowering people to choose one area of care over another, giving more choice and flexibility should be a benefit in this situation. If a patient is not comfortable in reporting abuse, they should still be able to refuse certain methods of care, thus freeing them from the potentials of further abuse. Chenitz (1983) discovered that for many older people moving to a nursing home placement was very stressful and potentially threatening. If experience of nursing homes have been negative then these individuals will become more isolated and increase their vulnerability within that particular setting. They need to be able to master this event in a positive way to enable them to deal with living in a nursing home life and thrive (Chenitz 1983).

Scenario for reflection

Imagine you are working in a care home and you observe a colleague mistreating a resident.
Imagine you are working for a private home agency and you observe a colleague mistreating an older person in their own home.
What action would you take?
What policies are in place to promote non-abusive behaviour?
Who would you talk to and what procedures would you follow in both scenarios?

From powerlessness to empowerment

The above phrase features in almost every article or book written about the abused older person – and not without reason. The phrase is probably best-placed to capture the sense that practitioners working with vulnerable older people invariably nurture: that the best amelioration or intervention they can offer is the regaining of self-determination by a vulnerable older person. Recent policy initiatives have accordingly attempted to give citizens greater choice in the services and care they can expect from professionals. This is evident in the 2005 Adult Social Care Green Paper, *Independence, Well-being and Choice* (DoH 2005a) in whose preface the then Secretary of State, John Reid said:

> We want to give individuals and their families and friends greater control over the way in which social care supports their needs. We want to support individuals to live as independently as possible for as long as possible.
>
> (2005a: 6)

This philosophy is looked upon favourably by many, yet in the case of the vulnerable adult judgements as to how they are supported in many instances devolved not from state to individual but to the individual's family who may seek to make care decisions for them. By contrast, direct payments and Individual and Personal Budgets are ways of financially empowering the older person and ensuring a degree of individual autonomy. Many older people now have personalized budgets to purchase services that will enable them to lead more independent lives. However, for some people they may be reliant on a carer or family member to claim these benefits and budgets for them. As the shift of care from in-house provision of services has moved to people being increasingly cared for in their own home, is the funding being used in the most appropriate way? Does the vulnerable adult have a voice when it comes to utilizing their payments? Alcock et al. (2010) recognize that the number of people receiving social care purchased by local authorities is decreasing, claiming that it is the most needy who are receiving far more intense support. How have the most needy been assessed? If social services are not putting in services for the remainder of the 'needy' population then it would appear that many private agencies are taking on this responsibility.

Stricter controls are now in place to protect the vulnerable adult and employers are now eligible to ask for enhanced disclosures with a barred-list check on anyone they are taking on in regulated activity. However, new employees and those changing jobs in regulated activity do not need to start applying for Independent Safeguarding Authority registration until July 2010 and Independent Safeguarding Authority registration does not become mandatory for these workers until November 2010. All other staff will be phased into the scheme from 2011. It is imperative that the vulnerable older person is made aware of these regulations so that they will be alerted to the fact that not all agency workers will have gone through the vetting and barring scheme until 2011. All employers have a legal duty to report to the Independent

Safeguarding Authority any member of staff they suspect of causing harm to vulnerable adults. The overriding aim of the Independent Safeguarding Authority will be to help avoid harm, or risk of harm, to vulnerable adults by preventing those who are deemed unsuitable to work with vulnerable adults from gaining access to them through their work.

Scenario for reflection

An older person living at home wants to employ a private agency to come in to their home to assist with daily chores.
What regulations are in place to protect the older person in such a context?
What advice would you give to them regarding employing such a person?

Strategies and mechanisms for coping with abuse

The state plays an important role in the protection of members of the public from harm – before harm has happened and after it has happened. The government see their role as advisors and enabling people at risk to become empowered. People are encouraged to make decisions based on informed choice. Many of the Department of Health documents support this view: *Our Health, Our Care, Our Say* (DoH 2006) is one in particular that actively encourages people to make decisions based on informed choice. The overall philosophy is one of encouragement and empowerment. If people are free to make their own choices, then they must also take responsibility when their choice does not work out to their satisfaction. Should a decision make a person more vulnerable, they must then be encouraged to look at alternative choices, once again empowering them to make a decision but not allowing them to wallow in self-pity and blame. The message is to make people realize that to cope in a vulnerable situation may result in some questioning their own decisions and self-belief.

It has been recognized through a number of research studies (Ogg and Bennett 1992; O'Keefe et al. 2007; Cooper et al. 2008; Action on Elder Abuse 2009) that vulnerable adults have the potential to fall prey to yet other forms of abuse. Moser (1998: 3) suggests that 'the more assets people have the less vulnerable they are, and the greater the erosion of people's assets, the greater their insecurity'. This notion of assets is most helpfully understood not only in terms of economic productivity and physical investments but also in terms of less immediately tangible guises. The assets may be those of knowledge, or contribution to family or community life. Society has a duty to promote the older person's assets, recognizing them as attributes and not something to hide from. Older people need to be encouraged to question and challenge, and not fear, retribution because of this. It is thought that when people are socially disadvantaged or lack political voice, their vulnerability is exacerbated further and that many of the causes of vulnerability are lack of access to information and knowledge, lack of public awareness, limited access to political power and representation (Aysan 1993). This suggests that to be vulnerable is complex and multifaceted. As a result vulnerability may not always be easily recognizable. Services need to be more responsive to people's needs, taking into account those vulnerable users. Cree and Myers (2008) suggest that if user empowerment is to have meaning, then practitioners need to consider how their policies and practices enable service users to be at the heart of planning and delivery, rather than an afterthought. Nolan et al.'s (2006) 'model of senses' embraces this philosophy and encourages involvement of the older person, as well as staff and carers, at all times. The 'senses' framework enables people to experience a sense of:

- security – to feel safe within relationships;
- belonging – to feel part of things;
- continuity – to experience links and consistency;
- purpose – to have a personally valuable goal or goals;
- achievement – to make progress towards a desired goal or goals;
- significance – to feel that you matter.

On similar lines, Barr and Hashagen (2007) have developed a ladder of empowerment. The steps on this ladder can be utilized with the vulnerable older person to ensure that they are given every opportunity to be empowered. The steps on the ladder involve:

- manipulation – to educate the individual, creating an element of participation;
- informing – telling people what is planned;
- consultation – offering options and listening to feedback;
- deciding together – encouraging others to provide additional ideas and join in decisions about the best way forward;
- acting together – deciding together and forming partnerships to act;
- supporting independent community interests – helping others to do what they want.

Both of these paradigms provide helpful conceptual tools for thinking about our practice in supporting at risk older people. Working with the older vulnerable person requires skilful communication, acts of diplomacy, and most importantly, a willingness to take seriously any complaint that may be mentioned. The *Simple Mistakes Shatter Lives Campaign* (HSE 2009) encourages and promotes intervention by those working with vulnerable people, in the hope that actions of those working with them may be taken to prevent any form of accident happening.

Partnerships

In 2005 the Department of Health launched their policy, *Partnerships for Older People* (POPPS; DoH 2005b). This was aimed at promoting the health, well-being and independence of the older person. It takes account of the safeguarding aspects of protection, justice and empowerment which are aimed at giving the older person power to make choices and decisions to benefit their well-being. With the advent of partnerships and social enterprise organizations, safeguarding must take a priority to ensure that all people who will be working in any regulated or controlled activity with vulnerable older groups will be scrutinized. The Independent Safeguarding Authority work in partnership with the Criminal Records Bureau (CRB) to gather this information, and people wishing to work with vulnerable older people will be asked to pay a fee, whereas the volunteers are not required to pay a registration fee. This should not be a cause for concern as the volunteers will have gone through a Criminal Record Bureau screening. This in itself will demonstrate commitment to working with this group of people.

As a result of the Partnerships for Older People (POPPS) safeguarding partnerships have been set up across the country and this involves professionals from a variety of areas working together to promote safeguarding in the older person. In January 2009 an example of this partnership was very evident as a group of professionals, namely social workers, police officers, nurses, housing officers, lawyers and voluntary and sector workers all responded to the consultation on *Safeguarding Adults: The Review of the No Secrets Guidance*. This is a very positive move towards future effective partnership working. Partnership working in Canada is extremely pro-active towards promoting and empowering older people. Empowerment groups have been set up whereby older people are trained to stand up for themselves and become knowledgeable about their rights (Brookman et al. 1996) Possibly the UK could take this as a benchmark of good practice and set up a similar scheme in the UK.

Scenario for reflection

You want to set up a safeguarding group in your area of work.
Who would you get involved in this?

What would be the purpose of this group?
How often would you meet?
How would you evaluate the success of this group?

Conclusion

As a result of the findings of the *No Secrets* review and subsequent policy initiatives there is a considerably heightened awareness of the risks to which vulnerable older adults are exposed (Sumner 2002). Multi-agency policies and procedures to protect vulnerable adults from abuse offer assistance to a variety of abusive situations – physical, sexual, psychological, financial and discriminatory. However, Action on Elder Abuse (2009) recognizes that there is still great variation in the support that vulnerable adults receive. Practitioners must ensure that highly trained individuals with relevant expertise in working with vulnerable adults have the skills to identify instances of abuse and take independent decisions to prevent unsuitable people gaining access to the vulnerable. Phil Hope, the Care Services Minister, said in response to the Action on Elder Abuse (2009) findings, that the policy context for working with at-risk adults increasingly recognizes that 'abuse of vulnerable adults is absolutely unacceptable and the government are deter-mined to improve safeguarding systems and the quality of life for people at risk of harm'.

For the initial moves in this direction to become systematically embedded, there needs to be more specialized education and training for formal and informal caregivers who are working and caring for vulnerable older people. There also needs to be further structural, cultural and attitudinal changes in society in order to prevent exploitation of the vulnerable older person. Ultimately, the best paradigm for working with at-risk older people is one which takes full cognisance not only of their vulnerabilities but also of their potentialities. Laslett (1989) in his seminal work regarding old age ('third age') referred to the fact that the longevity of the population would increase and that this was a great achievement to be enjoyed and celebrated. Laslett actively encouraged this development and proactiveness of later life. This approach is to be embraced as this attitude is the aspiration for many vulnerable older people who are working towards improving their lives. Members of society who are working with this group of people are in a privileged position in assisting older people to lead a fulfilled old age without fear.

Reflection on practice

Look around you at the many older people with whom you are in contact. Does their experience appear to conform to the following aspirations about well-being as an older person?

- Age should carry an element of respect.
- Age may mean being looked after.
- Age brings humour as life is looked back on with laughter and fun.
- Age should not mean isolation.
- Age should not bring crime into the home.
- Age should not bring fear.

References

Action on Elder Abuse (2007). Briefing paper: The UK study of abuse and neglect of older people. London: Action on Elder Abuse.

Action on Elder Abuse (2008) *A Study of the Effectiveness of Arrangements to Safeguard Adults from Abuse*. London: Commission for Social Care Inspection.

Action on Elder Abuse (2009) *Response to the Consultation on the Review of No Secrets*. London: Action on Elder Abuse.

Alcock, C., Daly, G. and Griggs, E. (2010) *Introducing Social Policy*. Harlow: Pearson Longman.

Aysan, Y.F. (1993) Keynote paper: vulnerability assessment. In P. Merriman and C. Browitt (eds) *Natural Disasters: Protecting Vulnerable Communities*: Proceedings of the Conference held in London, 13–15 October 1993. London: Royal Society.

Barr, A. and Hashagen, S. (2007) *Working with ABCD: Experience, Lessons and Issues from Practice*. London: Community Development Fund.

Brookman, L., Miller, N. and Nahmiash, D. (1996) *Standing up for Yourself: Empowerment Groups for the Elderly*. Poster Session. Quebec: Canadian Association on Gerontology.

Bytheway, B. (1995) *Ageism*. Buckingham: Open University Press.

Chambers, R. (1989) Vulnerability, coping and policy. *IDS Bulletin*, 20(2): 1–7.

Chenitz, W. (1983) Entry into a nursing home as status passage: a theory to guide nursing practice. *Geriatric Nursing*, 4(2): 92–7.

Commission on Integration and Cohesion (2007) *Research Papers*. London: Commission on Integration and Cohesion.

Cooper, C., Selwood, A. and Livingston, G. (2008) The prevalence of elder abuse and neglect: a systematic. *Age and Ageing*, 37(2): 151–60.

Cree, V. and Myers, S. (2008) *Social Work: Making a Difference*. Bristol: Policy.

Department for Children, Schools and Families (DCSF) (2009) *The Standards Fund 2008–2011*. Cheshire: Public Communications Unit.

Department of Health (DoH) (2000) *No Secrets Guidance*. London: The Stationery Office.

Department of Health (DoH) (2001) *National Service Framework for the Older Person*. London: The Stationery Office.

Department of Health (DoH) (2002) *National Service Framework for the Older Person-Supporting Implementation: Intermediate Care: Moving Forward*. London: The Stationery Office.

Department of Health (DoH) (2005a) *Independence, Well-being and Choice*. London: The Stationery Office.

Department of Health (DoH) (2005b) *Partnerships for Older People*. London: The Stationery Office.

Department of Health (DoH) (2006) *Our Health, Our Care, Our Say*. London: The Stationery Office.

Department of Health (DoH) (2008) *Safeguarding Adults: A Consultation on the Review of the 'No Secrets' Guidance*. London: Department of Health.

Department of Health (DoH) (2009) *National Dementia Strategy*. London: The Stationery Office.

Department of Health (DoH) (2010) *Written Ministerial Statement. Government Response to the Consultation on Safeguarding Adults: The Review of the No Secrets Guidance*. London: Department of Health.

Department of Health/Comic Relief (2007) *Action on Elder Abuse*. London: Department of Health.

Gosney, M. (2009) The vulnerable elderly. *Pulse Clinical*, October.

Health and Safety Executive (HSE) (2009) *Simple Mistakes Can Shatter Lives*, London: HSE.

Help the Aged (2006) *Hidden Voices: Older People's Experiences of Abuse*, Executive Summary. London.

Hope, P. (2010) Written ministerial statement: Government response to the Consultation on safeguarding adults. The review of the No Secrets Guidance. London: Department of Health.

Kelly, F. (2010) Abusive interactions: research in locked wards for people with dementia. *Social Policy & Society*, 9(2): 267–77.

Laslett, P. (1989) *A Fresh Map of Life: The Emergence of the Third Age*. London: Weidenfeld & Nicholson.

McAlpine, C. (2008) Elder abuse and neglect. *Age & Ageing*, 37(2): 132–33.

McCreadie, C. et al. (2006) First steps: the UK National Prevalence Study of the mistreatment and abuse of older people. *Journal of Adult Protection*, 8(3): 4–11.

Moser, C. (1998) The asset-vulnerability framework: reassessing urban poverty reduction strategies. *World Development*, 26(1): 1–19.

Mowlan, A. et al. (2007) *UK Study of Abuse and Neglect of Older People: Qualitative Findings*. London: Comic Relief and Department of Health.

Nahmiash, D. (2000) From powerlessness to empowerment. In J. Pritchard (ed.) *Elder Abuse Work: Best Practice in Britain and Canada*. London: Jessica Kingsley.

Nolan, M., Brown, J., Davies, S., Nolan, J. and Keady, J. (2006) The senses framework: improving care for older people through a relationship-centred approach. *Getting Research into Practice* (GRiP) Report No. 2, Sheffield: University of Sheffield.

Ogg, J. and Bennett, G. (1992) Elder abuse in Britain. *British Medical Journal*, 305: 998–9.

O'Keefe, M., et al. (2007) *UK Study of Abuse and Neglect of Older People: Prevalence Survey Report*. London: National Centre for Social Research.

Pritchard, J. (2000) *Elder Abuse Work: Best Practice in Britain and Canada*. London: Jessica Kinsgley.

Reed, J., Stanley, D. and Clarke, C. (2004) *Health, Well-Being and Older People*. Bristol: Policy.

Sumner, K. (2002) *No Secrets: The Protection of Vulnerable Adults from Abuse: Local Codes of Practice – Findings from an Analysis of Local Codes of Practice*. London: Centre for Policy on Ageing.

Turner, B. (2006) *Vulnerability and Human Rights*. Philadelphia, PA: State University Press.

Linking theory with practice examples

Agnes Fanning and Roger Dalrymple

The previous chapters have demonstrated many of the recent government initiatives and legislative safeguards that are available to support the at-risk adult in a variety of circumstances. It will be clear to the reader that the categories of 'adults at risk' investigated in the preceding chapters are not exhaustive. For, as we have seen, vulnerability is not a stable state and different individuals may traverse, or find themselves isolated within, different domains of risk across the life-span. While the foregoing chapters have tended to emphasize individual risk domains such as 'physical disability', 'mental health' and 'the older person', it will be clear to the reader that in many scenarios where a practitioner is working with an at-risk adult, the individual in question will be situated within more than one risk domain – with the prospect of entering still further risk domains in the future if positive intervention and support are not forthcoming.

Many at-risk adults need support to gain some form of independence and, as explored in a number of the preceding chapters, some people are not even aware that they are vulnerable, or are reluctant to be categorized as 'at risk'. This can make identification and amelioration of need difficult to deal with in an effective manner. How can the practitioner identify those instances where different domains of risk coincide? How can the practitioner anticipate those areas of risk that may arise in the future for a service user, client or patient with whom they are working?

To aid the beginning and developing practitioner in meeting these challenges, Part Two of this book presents four sustained case studies of working with adults at risk of harm. In each case study, one risk domain is apparently salient (be it substance misuse, sexual orientation, insecure accommodation, migration), but it will transpire in more than one of these case-studies how different risk domains overlap and how the informed practitioner must recognize this intersectionality of risk and adjust their practice accordingly.

Working through these case studies, or treating them as the basis for class or workshop discussion, will provide the beginning and developing practitioner with concrete demonstration of the concepts, theories and models of risk and exclusion that have been discussed in the previous chapters. The case studies will enable readers to reflect on challenging and complex situations where risk and vulnerability are not always obvious, not entirely predictable, and where creative and effective interventions require our compassion, empathy and detailed understanding.

PART 2
Case Studies and Practice Examples

9 Culture, identity, disability, addiction – multiple domains of risk

Jo Edwards

This case study analyses a social work intervention designed to assist an individual whose situation and experiences exposed him to multiple domains of risk: physical disability, homelessness, alcohol dependency, offending and disadvantaged cultural identity within UK society. The case study spans approximately three years of intervention and will also provide a theoretical perspective on some of the issues underpinning the complexity of presenting 'needs'. It is written as a social worker's 'journey' of involvement. It is not intended to be a paragon of 'good practice' but rather a reflection on the competing demands of meeting a range of complex needs within a service bound by legislative and resource limitations within social work practice. This is a historical narrative in relation to the service user of the local-authority Physical and Sensory Disability Team, as intervention began in 2005 and ended in 2008. Some fundamental changes in Department of Health guidance and regulations have taken place since this case study was completed.

The following case study aims to provide social care practitioners and social workers with a brief overview of working with complex and multiple needs. It will illustrate ways in which such work may be managed by taking a holistic approach to ameliorating needs and risks, in partnership with the service user and other relevant agencies. The study will reflect how complex needs promote complex risks, and these can be compounded by multiple exclusion, discrimination and structural oppression. Substance misuse/abuse, mental health, physical disability and race/ethnicity are all strands of societal and structural oppression which need to be taken into account as separate, but interlinked, experiences of disadvantage.

CASE STUDY 'CHARACTERS'[1]

Carlton   Service user of Physical and Sensory Disability Team
Mary   Service user of Community Learning Disability Team

Introducing Carlton

Carlton is a 46-year-old man, who describes his ethnicity as Black Jamaican. Carlton has a diagnosis of cerebral palsy, which affects his legs and lower back and he requires a walking aid. He also has a diagnosis of epilepsy for which he is required to take medication. Carlton is in receipt of welfare benefits. He is time-disorientated and has difficulty managing his personal care. He uses cannabis lightly and is alcohol dependent – he drinks up to 20 litres of cider a day. Carlton has a history of offending and has been discharged into the community from prison following a six-month sentence for threatening a bus driver with a knife.

Carlton lives in a housing association flat but he is not a tenant. His 'landlady', Mary, holds the tenancy and she is a service user of the Community Learning Disability Team. Mary has a mild learning disability, poor health, and is also alcohol dependent. She has been served with several anti-social behaviour orders, and has demonstrated verbal and physical aggressive behaviour towards others, though she has not been convicted. Carlton does not pay any rent to Mary, but instead provides her with alcohol. He also makes use of Mary's laundry service which is provided by the local authority.

Carlton and Mary frequently experience discriminatory abuse within the community. They have had the windows of the flat broken with bricks and fires set in the letterbox.

Beginning intervention

Involvement with Carlton began on referral from the Community Learning Disability Team with a request for assessment. The Community Learning Disability social worker providing professional support to Mary had become concerned about a recent decline in Carlton's health, and the growing disputes involving physical and verbal abuse between Carlton and Mary.

Learning point

The key legislation for assessment of adults with physical and sensory disability is the National Health Service and Community Care Act (NHSCCA) 1990 – Section 47: 'Where it appears to a local authority that any person for whom they provide

> or arrange for the provision of community care services may be in need of any
> such services, the authority –
>
> (a) shall carry out an assessment of his needs for those services; and
> (b) having regard to the results of that assessment, shall then decide whether his
>   needs call for the provision by them of any such services'.

The purpose of the initial visit with Carlton was to complete a community care assessment. Carlton presented as disengaged and did not wish to discuss his 'care needs'.

The initial barrier

It could be argued that the focus of the assessment can act as a restriction on the interaction between service user and worker. The assessment 'tool' is concerned with *medical* diagnosis and works by defining lack of 'ability'. Marks (1999) suggests that this medical model views disability as personal 'damage' or dysfunction, requiring diagnosis and treatment by a professional. Additionally, Ryan (1971) believes that focusing on disability at the individual or personal level further creates an example of blaming the victim.

'Care management' is a term used to define the process of assessment, service provision and review. The process could be argued to reinforce the medical model and further increase the level of oppression experienced by people with disabilities. The National Health Service and Community Care Act 1990 places a duty on local authorities to carry out an assessment of need where it appears that a person may be in need of services (S47(1)(a) NHSCCA 1990).

The term 'need' may have negative connotations for service users. While social workers are exhorted to focus on 'needs', the issue of 'rights' becomes less explicit, as does the issue of user-led assessment. Also, 'need' can imply 'neediness' which, in contemporary society's ideology of consumerism and individualism, is perceived negatively. Dalrymple and Burke (2007) argue that practitioners, while working from an anti-oppressive perspective, must ensure that the rights of service users are not infringed. Additionally, the General Social Care Council (GSCC) *Code of Practice* places responsibility on social care workers to protect and promote the rights and interests of service users and carers.

Banks (2006) suggests that social services departments are bureaucratic in nature, and essentially exist to provide services in an impartial manner. This expectation of impartiality is required of social work practitioners, but conflict and personal resonance will most likely occur as the social worker is involved in the service user's personal struggles and pain. It would be an exceptionally 'detached' social worker who could complete an assessment of need without a fundamental empathic understanding of the humanity of a given situation.

Engagement

Several more visits with Carlton ensued before he agreed to completion of an overview assessment. During these visits, Carlton began to engage positively, and a rapport began to be established with the practitioner. It was, however, essential to remain goal-centred in order to remain focused on 'the task in hand'. Without completion of assessment, access to services is prevented. Laborde (1994) outlines a five-step approach to goal-centred communication. These steps include aiming for a specific outcome, keeping positive, 'tuning in' to the other person, trying to reach agreed goals and then working out both short- and long-term objectives.

Short-term goals

The main objective following assessment was short-term risk prevention or minimization. Carlton was assessed to be at 'critical' risk for activities of daily living under the Fair Access to Care Services (FACS) eligibility criteria, 2003 (now superseded by 'Prioritizing Need in the Context of Putting People First', 2010). Carlton was assessed to be at risk of falls and also increasing ill-health due to lack of personal care/hygiene. Carlton was also potentially at financial risk as he was unclear about his benefit receipt.

The first of the three short-term goals identified, therefore, was to organize a full benefits check. Novak (1996) states that poverty not only serves as a barrier to ownership and material possession, but it also delimits a person's place, position and relationship within and relative to society. The consequences of poverty become further compounded when linked to other forms of systemic oppression, such as 'race' and disablism (Becker and MacPherson 1988).

The second short-term risk management proposal was to make adaptations to the property (bars and 'grab' handles) to minimize risk of falls. Carlton agreed to these, but did not wish to have assistance with personal care. A complaint had, at this time, come in from the local authority's laundry service about Carlton using Mary's service, and it was important that he had his own service in order to prevent Mary from losing hers.

Long-term goals

Carlton's alcohol dependency was contributing to increasingly poor health and mobility issues. The long-term objective was to address the issue of alcohol dependency, and Carlton was open to discussion about this and also to looking at possible treatment.

There were ongoing safeguarding concerns with regard to the abusive relationship between Carlton and Mary. There was evident risk to workers due to the level of alcohol consumption and resulting behaviour, thus a 'two-handed' visit was essential. Other professionals involved with Carlton and Mary were the police and the domestic violence unit and they too followed this policy.

According to Penrod (1983), anti-social aggression is any behaviour which, with intention, results in either physical or psychological harm to an individual. Frustration can make people angry, but angry people do not always behave aggressively. Hull and Bond (1986) found that violence is increased by the consumption of alcohol, and it has been well documented that alcohol interferes with typical cognitive functioning (Taylor and Sears 1988).

There is evidence that nearly all addictions are represented to a higher degree in men than in women, but there are cultural variations (Zilberman et al. 2003; see further Chapter 7). Langeland et al. (2003) have identified that being subject to abuse as a child is strongly linked to the development of addiction, as is an individual's propensity towards anti-social behaviour, anxiety and depression.

Learning point

According to the International Classification of Diseases-10 (WHO 1992), at least three of the following characteristics must have been experienced or exhibited at some time during the previous year for an individual to be classified as 'addicted'.

- Difficulties in controlling substance-taking behaviour in terms of its onset, termination, or levels of use.
- A strong desire or sense of compulsion to take the substance.
- Progressive neglect of alternative pleasures or interests because of psychoactive substance use, increased amount of time necessary to obtain or take the substance or to recover from its effects.
- Persisting with substance use despite clear evidence of overtly harmful consequences, depressive mood states consequent to heavy use, or drug-related impairment of cognitive functioning.
- Evidence of tolerance, such that increased doses of the psychoactive substance are required in order to achieve effects originally produced by lower doses.

- A physiological withdrawal state when substance use has ceased or been reduced, as evidenced by the characteristic withdrawal syndrome for the substance or use of the same (or close related) substance with the intention of relieving or avoiding withdrawal symptoms.

Although Carlton had a 'roof over his head', his situation defined him as legally 'homeless' (see further Chapter 6 on insecure accommodation).

Learning point

The legal definition of homelessness for England and Wales can be found in the 1996 Housing Act: 'A person is homeless if:
There is no accommodation that they are entitled to occupy;
or
They have accommodation but it is not reasonable for them to continue to occupy this accommodation'.

Carolton had no rights to tenancy and could be evicted at any time by Mary. He had access to a sofa and kept this for himself by ensuring that Mary had a continual supply of alcohol. According to Seal (2007) people who are homeless are often perceived as people who are difficult to work with. This is mainly due to the fact they do not conform to existing services, and are then seen to become a 'problem'. Seal (2005) advises that the people who experience a number of serious, sometimes life-threatening illnesses and who are also homeless often have overwhelming difficulties to manage.

Carlton himself advised that he was uneasy with his current housing situation – a positive development since, according to Bateman (2000), any action taken on behalf of a service user should start, and end, with that service user directing the intervention. This is one of the main principles of advocacy. Assisting Carlton to gain access to a secure tenancy was, therefore, a second long-term goal. The fact that it would not be resolved more promptly became apparent when the local housing association refused initially to offer Carlton sheltered accommodation due to the high volume of police activity within Mary's house, the number of complaints made by residents within the neighbourhood and his level of alcohol consumption.

The issue became even more complicated when the housing association advised that Mary would have to evict him 'formally' (which she was not prepared to do because she would lose access to alcohol).

Carlton's history as told by Carlton

Carlton stated that he was born in Jamaica to a very young woman, who, after Carlton's birth, moved to the UK leaving him in the care of his maternal grandmother. Carlton continued to be raised by his grandmother until she died when he was aged eleven. He was then sent to the UK to be reunited with his mother who was unable to provide a home for him. He was then placed in a residential children's home in the east end of London.

Carlton describes this period of his life as particularly traumatic. He had very little spoken English when he arrived in the UK, and no understanding of the culture, social norms and expectations of British society. It could be suggested that Carlton would have experienced loss and bereavement in terms of his grandmother's death – and this was possibly compounded by his perceived rejection by his birth mother following his entry to the UK. Carlton described his experience of racism when entering the UK and how this became entrenched, with his perception of his disability, within his self-concept. According to Macpherson (1999), covert racism can prove as damaging to an individual as its more overt forms.

Carlton stated he was placed in a foster home aged 16 after his placement with the residential children's home concluded. He advised that he became drug- and alcohol-dependent and began offending during this time.

It transpired over time that Carlton had 98 previous convictions, many of which were convictions of actual and grievous bodily harm. His first offence, as a juvenile, was manslaughter. Although Carlton does not have a diagnosis of mental ill-health, he had a psychiatric report (convened by the court) which investigated his statement that he had heard voices telling him to 'kill couples'. The report concluded that this was as a result of heavy alcohol and cannabis use.

Carlton stated that his disability was unacceptable to him – that it meant he was not 'normal' and that he 'couldn't bear to see his reflection in shop windows'. He advised that he used alcohol in order to feel 'normal – like everyone else'.

Learning point

According to Stone (2005) 'cultural competence' (the knowledge and understanding of the potential impact of particular cultural values on identity) continues

> to develop importance within all front line service provision due to the increasingly diverse populations in western cultural societies. This is particularly relevant within services for people with disabilities as the norms and values of that person's culture may impact on self-belief, self-esteem and self-efficacy.

Evil spirits, ghosts, duppies and sin

Jamaican society holds entrenched belief systems about disability. Disability is seen as a punishment for 'wrongdoing' and the causes may be 'evil spirits, ghosts, duppies, *obeah*, or *guzu* as well as natural causes' (Leavitt 1992; Heinz and Payne-Jackson 1997). *Obeah* or *guzu* is a belief in the ability to harness supernatural forces for good and evil, health or sickness. There still exists a notion among the 'educated classes' and professionals that disability is a result of sin.

It is believed that the punishment for this 'sin' may be visited on the perpetrator, or the perpetrator's offspring in the form of a disability. Therefore, disability can give rise to intense feelings of shame and guilt. It is not unusual for a child with a congenital birth 'defect' to be hidden from public view for life, or for a mother to openly reject her child. Carlton advised that he 'had no father'. Illegitimacy is often a source of derision in Jamaican culture.

Although Carlton was extremely reluctant to talk about his early years, it was apparent from what he said that he was extremely attached to his grandmother. It is possible that Carlton's mother rejected him on grounds of his disability and his possible illegitimacy, and that he had little contact with Jamaican society as he may have been kept 'out of sight' in his grandmother's care.

Carlton's self-belief

It is necessary to consider how Jamaican cultural beliefs may have shaped Carlton's early, formative years and his existing self-identity. Wijsen (1999) believes that culture is a 'meaning system' which is shared by members of a group in order to interpret ideas and for behavioural organization. This system of meanings includes ideas about the self, or identity. Thompson (2001) explores the power of 'culture' in forming our opinions and beliefs. Berger (1996) believes our own consciousness is structured by the structures of society and that it penetrates beyond the surface, being more than that which envelops us.

If Carlton's own self-beliefs were shaped by Jamaican cultural belief, then he may have felt that he was being punished for his own, or his ancestor's 'sins'. This is likely to have compounded his feelings of needing to be 'normal' and his reluctance to have his disability acknowledged.

Hall (1990) believes that identity is always in a process of development, and never becomes an accomplished state of being. If this is the case, Carlton's identity has been, and is being, shaped not just by Jamaican cultural beliefs, but also by western cultural perspectives on disability. In western culture, 'disablism' is described by Thompson (2001: 111) as 'systematic discrimination and prejudice against people with disabilities which produces a milieu of oppression and degradation'.

Our sense of self-worth has a very powerful effect on emotional states such as liking or disliking ourselves: depression can cause feelings of worthlessness. In relation to substance addiction, motivation to change can be decreased due to a devaluation of one's own sense of lack of worth. This means an individual would be less likely to abstain or cease activities that cause self-harm. In some cases, substances that 'numb' feelings or increase confidence are likely to be perceived as rewarding by someone with low self-esteem (West and Shiffman 2004). Gaultney et al. (1999) suggests that fatigue – both in the physical and mental sense (including depressed mood) – is likely to inhibit thought and action and thereby disallow recovery.

The drink agenda

Following successful intervention in terms of Community Occupational Therapy mobility aids, benefits check – and a resultant increase in Disability Living Allowance – and also a local authority laundry service, Carlton requested assistance with his use of alcohol, and appeared adamant that he wanted to live a life 'free from addiction'. With Carlton's consent the Community Drug and Alcohol Services (CDAS) was contacted.

The CDAS social worker presented Carlton to a CDAS panel for funding for residential placement. Two issues were raised, the first being that funding is only agreed if a service user has demonstrated 'motivation' through attending a community-based counselling service, and the second that service provision was likely to be extremely limited due to Carlton's needs in relation to his mobility issues.

The community-based counselling service was not currently available to Carlton due to staff shortages. Indeed, had the service been available, there are some doubts about Carlton's ability to engage due to his limited mobility. Here again lies demonstration that Carlton's diagnosis and aptitude will possibly increase his vulnerability to becoming socially isolated. Indeed, a review of a recent list of rehabilitation units available in the UK published in *Drink and Drugs News*[2] reveals that out of 166 units, only two explicitly mention provision for people with limited mobility – the approach necessary for Carlton.

Two presentations at panel, spanning three months, were necessary for funding to be agreed. After approximately six months, an 'out of county' placement was identified as meeting his complex needs, and which offered community rehabilitation after an 18-month programme. After six weeks, Carlton requested a return.

Kearney and O'Sullivan (2003) propose that there needs to be a positive change in self-perception during the process of change of behaviour. They describe this as a stage of 'critical reappraisal of self and situation'. If the positive change is constrained, however, by a lack of commitment to the new identity (e.g. a 'non-drinker'), or by negative old beliefs about self then it is likely that a permanent change in behaviour (abstinence) is unlikely to be achieved. There were concerns, following the rehabilitation report, that Carlton's emotional needs were left unmet following his medical 'detox'. Carlton's physical mobility decreased in the aftermath of detox and he required the use of a wheelchair. He was not offered individual counselling at this stage, and the unit stated that they had not been able to offer him a private room, as promised, due to the fact that they had made an error in booking. This meant that Carlton remained under supervision within the detox 'ward', was without privacy but in the company of several other service users undergoing detox programmes. Carlton was not prepared to consider a rehabilitation programme again during my involvement with him.

A new home

While liaising with the rehabilitation centre, there was also continuing dialogue with the local housing association.

> ### Learning point
>
> Evidence suggests that individuals representing black and minority ethnic groups are overrepresented as at risk of homelessness as a result of living in 'poor quality housing in run-down neighbourhoods which can be blighted by racist harassment and crime. Academic studies indicate that three times as many black and minority ethnic households present as homeless compared with other households' (DoH 2002).

The issues presenting for Carlton in terms of assistance with housing were complex due to the level of verbal and physical aggression between him and Mary, and the frequency of police intervention. The housing association stated concern with regard to Carlton's history of offending and maintained that due to his ongoing 'behaviour', Carlton was making himself 'intentionally homeless', a state (on which see further Chapter 6) which can be determined under the following criteria (among others):

- where someone is evicted because of anti-social behaviour such as nuisance to neighbours, harassment etc.;
- where someone is evicted because of violence or threats of violence by them towards an associated person (Housing Act 1996).

The housing association argued that even though Carlton was considered to be legally homeless, the fact that he was staying in 'temporary' accommodation need not be considered to break the link with 'intentional homelessness' (Housing Act 1996).

In order to promote the opportunity for a safe and reasonable housing opportunity for Carlton it was necessary to engage in professional advocacy support on his behalf with the housing association. According to Bateman (2000), advocacy is centred on the rights of service users. He argues that advocacy brings a perspective to individual work which is centred on rights, and can prevent the service user experiencing, or feeling, blame for situations beyond the control of the service user.

Multi-professional engagement clarified that the aggressive behaviour between Carlton and Mary was inter-dependent. It was, therefore, argued that by ensuring Carlton was offered another housing opportunity, this would cease.

Legally Carlton could be considered for 'priority need' for housing. According to the Housing Act (1996), applicants should be considered under the following conditions (among others):

> a person who is vulnerable as a result of old age, mental illness or handicap or physical disability or other special reason, or with whom such a person resides or might reasonably be expected to reside.

Carlton was successfully offered 'warden-assisted' accommodation which met his mobility issues, and professional support continued with regard to his ongoing health issues, including medication management of epilepsy and financial assistance in order to continue to secure tenancy. Carlton remains alcohol dependent.

Conclusion

The vulnerability of Carlton was evident throughout this case study and during this intervention there were many areas of complexity to manage and understand in order to provide the most effective services possible. These gave rise to some conflicts and dilemmas between professional and personal values.

Cultural competency allowed the worker to conceptualize some of the self-belief issues that Carlton may have been experiencing. An understanding of substance misuse, dependency and addiction developed and this allowed the worker to engage with the service user from an anti-discriminatory perspective. Acknowledging life-experience, and the potential impact on a person's behaviour (including offending) allowed the worker to gain an objective perspective of this service user as a 'whole' person, and to ensure that he was assisted to maximize his life opportunities. Ultimately, when working with adults, risk has to be considered in part as a matter of choice. This choice is made by the service user and although this choice can have an emotional impact on the worker, the detraction of choice will be an infringement on the individual's rights, independence and right to self-determination.

Notes

1   Pseudonyms have been assigned throughout this case study.
2   www.drinkanddrugs.net

References

Banks, S. (2006) *Ethics and Values in Social Work*, 3rd edn. London: Palgrave.

Bateman, N. (2000) *Advocacy Skills for Health and Social Care Professionals*. London: Jessica Kingsley.

Becker, S. and MacPherson, S. (eds) (1988) *Public Issues: Private Pain, Poverty, Social Work and Social Policy*. London: Social Services Insight Books.

Berger, M. (1996). *Cross-cultural Team Building: Guidelines for More Effective Communication and Negotiation*. London: McGraw-Hill.

Dalrymple, J. and Burke, S. (2007) *Anti-Oppressive Practice*, 2nd edn. Buckingham: Open University Press.

Department of Health (DoH) (2002) Homelessness Code of Guidance for Local Authorities. London: Office of the Deputy Prime Minister.

Gaultney, J.F., Kipp, K., Weinstein, J.A. and McNeill, J. (1999) Inhibition and mental effort in attention deficit hyperactivity disorder. *Journal of Developmental and Physical Disabilities*, 11: 105–14.

Hall, S. (1990) Cultural identity and diaspora. In J. Rutherford (ed.), *Identity, Community, Culture and Difference*. London: Lawrence and Wishart.

Heinz, A. and Payne-Jackson, A. (1997). Acculturation of explanatory models: Jamaican blood terms and concepts. *MACLAS Latin American Essays*, 11 (April): 19.

Hull, J. and Bond, C. (1986) Social and behavioral consequences of alcohol consumption and expectancy: a meta-analysis. *Psychological Bulletin*, 99: 347–60.

Kearney, M.H. and O'Sullivan, J. (2003) Identity shifts as turning points in health behaviour change. *Western Journal of Nursing Research*, 25: 134–52.

Laborde, G.Z. (1994) *Influencing with Integrity: Management Skills for Communication and Negotiation*. London: Crown.

Langeland, W., Draijer, N. and van den Brink, W. (2003) Assessment of lifetime physical and sexual abuse in treated alcoholics: validity of the Addiction Severity Index. *Addictive Behaviors*, 28(5): 871–81.

Leavitt, R.L. (1992). *Disability and Rehabilitation in Rural Jamaica. An Ethnographic Study*. Madison: Fairleigh Dickenson University Press.

Macpherson, Sir W. (1999) *The Stephen Lawrence Inquiry: Report of an Inquiry by Sir William Macpherson of Cluny*, CM 4262-I. London: Stationery Office, available online at: http://www.archive.official-documents.co.uk/document/cm42/4262/4262.htm

Marks, D. (1999) *Disability: Controversial Debates and Psychosocial Perspectives*. London: Routledge.

Novak, M. (1996) 'Poverty: facts and feelings'. *Druzboslovne razprave (Sociological Essays)*, 12: 22–23 (84–98).

Penrod, H. (1983) *Social Psychology*. Englewood Cliffs, NJ: Prentice-Hall.

Ryan, W. (1971) *Blaming the Victim*. London: Vintage.

Seal, M. (2005) *Resettling Homeless People: Theory and Practice*. Lyme Regis: Russell House.

Seal, M. (ed.) (2007) *Understanding and Responding to Homeless Experiences, Identities and Cultures*. Lyme Regis: Russell House.

Stone, J. (2005). *Culture and Disability: Providing Culturally Competent Services*. Thousand Oaks, CA: Sage.

Taylor, S.P. and Sears, J.D. (1988) The effects of alcohol and persuasive social pressure on human physical aggression. *Aggressive Behavior*, 14: 237–43.

Thompson, N. (2001) *Anti-Discriminatory Practice*, 3rd edn. Basingstoke: Palgrave.

West, R. and Shiffman, S. (2004) *Smoking Cessation*. Oxford: Health Press.

Wijsen, F. (1999) Beyond the fatal impact theory: globalization and its cultural underpinnings. In M. Amaladoss (ed.), *Globalization and Its Victims: As Seen by the Victims*. Delhi: Cambridge University Press, 122–31.

World Health Organization (1992) The ICD-10 Classification of Mental and Behavioural Disorders Clinical descriptions and diagnostic guidelines. Accessed online: www.who.int/entity/classifications/icd/en/bluebook.pdf

Zilberman, M.L., Tavares, H., Blume, S.B. and el-Guebaly, N. (2003) Substance use disorders: sex differences and psychiatric comorbidities. *Canadian Journal of Psychiatry*, 48(1): 5–15.

Further resources

Department of Health website, www.dh.gov.uk/en/index.htm
General Social Care website, www.gscc.org.uk

10 Sexual orientation

Lalage Harries

This case study takes a counsellor's perspective on sexual orientation as a risk domain and looks at the psychological impact of 'coming out' for three individuals and the factors that contained them or left them vulnerable. These experiences are highlighted as common and recurring themes in LGBTQ (lesbian, gay, bisexual, transgender, queer or questioning) vulnerability and exclusion, as demonstrated by recent research drawn on throughout the case study and by the knowledge of a practising counselling services manager for a long-running LGBT (lesbian, gay, bisexual or transgender) service interviewed for this study. While the bulk of available research concerns gay men and lesbians, the continuum of sexual identity and experience contains those not easily categorized, and often forgotten.

Names and some details of individuals have been altered to protect their anonymity.

Our sexuality can be invisible, denied and sidelined by the requirements and coercions of those around us, and by the expectations communicated from birth by wider society that we will be heterosexual and that this is the common, and by implication, 'normal' state of things. This can have a profoundly damaging effect on LGBTQ individuals,[1] as this case study explores, with particular reference to:

- hate crimes and current hate crime legislation;
- internalized homophobia;
- independence and multiple vulnerabilities;
- examples of good practice.

One of the pervasive themes of this case study is the impact on individuals of this cultural assumption that heterosexuality is key to the development of an integrated and secure sense of self. The impact of living in a society which automatically assumes that an individual is heterosexual will be starkly apparent when looking at the experiences of Cathy, Linda and Michael, the three subjects of our case study.

Cathy grew up on an army base in the north of England, the youngest in a family centred on the military. She reports being unaware of even the words 'gay' and 'lesbian' and their meanings, but recalls unnamed derision around lesbianism: 'I was always aware of the reaction in the house; like "ooh, Martina Navratilova's won Wimbledon again, isn't it about time a *woman* won it"'. The disjuncture between her unnamed inner (lesbian) world and the external 'hetero-assumptive' world (where normative heterosexuality is presumed rather than open to debate) left Cathy feeling that she might be 'seen through' and that 'at any moment the men in white coats might appear'. This strained not only her sense of normality but even sanity, and reinforced her belief that she must be silent about her feelings, leaving her excluded from any form of support.

Going to college provided her with both the role models which she had been lacking and the language to express herself; it also brought the conflict between her inner and outer worlds to a head. Cathy tentatively attempted to come out, choosing to test this with her stepfather, whose response – 'don't tell your mother, it'll kill her' – was endorsed by her siblings.

Her family were attempting to silence the part of her they found unacceptable; the weak sense of self she had developed in that environment made it hard for her to challenge them, leaving her torn between family acceptance and a powerful need to 'be authentic' which expressed itself physically: 'I used to wake up crying . . . just couldn't sleep [I felt] as if I had let myself down'. Severe insomnia, unexplained illness and falling grades in her studies continued during the two years she kept her sexuality secret from her mother at the behest of her wider family. During this time she became involved in heterosexual relations in an attempt to conform to normative expectations.

Cathy's vulnerability took on a new dimension when she became attracted to one of her lecturers and began to extricate herself from this heterosexual relationship. Uncertain of what she wanted, yet finding her sexuality increasingly impossible to hide, she sought to break away from her then boyfriend, whose response to her attempts to end the relationship included violence and repeated threats against her and her family.

Cathy's uncertainty as to whether the assault had a conscious homophobic element compounded her confusion and sense of responsibility for the situation that had now arisen. If her experience of growing up had taught her that heterosexuality represented psychological safety, in a very real sense, it now also represented *physical* safety. When she had been playing the heterosexual role 'correctly', she was safe; when the mask began to fall, she was in danger and found herself unsupported by social authority, as represented by the police, who did not support her in pressing charges after her partner's violence towards her.

Learning point

Hate crimes are defined by the Association of Chief Police Officers (ACPO) as 'any hate incident, which constitutes a criminal offence, perceived by the victim or any other person as being motivated by prejudice or hate'.

Stonewall, one of the largest LGBTQ pressure groups in the UK, conducted a 2008 survey of homophobic hate crime, finding that 'one in five lesbian and gay people have experienced a homophobic hate crime or incident in the last three years' (Dick 2008: 5), while 'half of all hate incidents reported to the police resulted in no action being taken other than it being recorded' (Dick 2008: 25).

The high prevalence of homophobic violence or harassment being experienced by LGBTQ people has serious implications for mental health and physical safety: 'Two thirds of those reporting hate incidents were not referred to or informed about any support or advice services available to them' (Dick 2008: 25). This is especially troubling as, through most of the country, those surveyed felt they were more likely to 'alter their behaviour so as not to appear gay' than to report an incident to the police (Dick 2008: 32).

Unsurprisingly, the survey also shows massive under-reporting of hate crimes, leaving victims unsupported.

Like many victims of crimes, Cathy felt a misplaced sense of guilt and responsibility for the threats made to her family. This tapped into the 'deep sense of self-loathing' Cathy described as part of the cumulative effect of years of homophobic feedback. Ultimately this undermined her ego and internalized negative associations with LGBTQ culture which proved hard to shake off, as demonstrated by her reaction to exposure to 'out' information sources.

'I was reading [a library book] at home and out slipped this piece of paper: "Sheffield Lesbian Line". At first I thought "No, no, no that's not me": I was horrified that this piece of paper would be in this book'.

Learning point

Internalized homophobia is the unconscious acceptance of homophobic views experienced by LGBTQ persons growing up and living in a hetero-assumptive culture.

According to a counselling services manager at London Friend, a service offering support, counselling and advice to the LGBTQ community in London, there is a 'high frequency of internalized homophobia' as a presenting issue among clients. Internalized homophobia is often a factor in anxiety, depression and other mental health issues among London Friend clients, 'which may cause lifelong vulnerability and (self) exclusion from support'.[2]

As our emerging identity develops, we want to see this reflected back positively to feel secure and accepted. If this is not received from family and community, LGBTQ role models in media and culture become even more crucial. All the more worrying is that 'four in five young lesbian and gay people have no access to any information at school about lesbian and gay issues' (Hunt and Jensen 2007: 10).

Increasing visibility of LGBTQ figures and news and improving access to information for young people is crucial to normalizing LGBTQ experience and combating homophobia. The Equality and Human Rights Commission reports: 'LGB lifestyles have remained largely invisible . . . [in British society] meaning that significant disadvantage and discrimination has gone unnoticed and remained unchallenged' (Equality and Human Rights Commission 2009: 6).

Some months after finding the information leaflet, Cathy contacted Sheffield Lesbian Line, an action which became a turning point for her. The service 'was cheap as chips because it was funded' and offered the alternative, lesbian community Cathy had never encountered before: 'it was such a relief, to have this place. There were teachers; there were writers, social workers – all sorts of people. They were successful, they were happy. It was such a revelation'.

With support, Cathy was in time able to develop a strong, confident identity as a lesbian and educate her family, who, in turn, now challenge homophobic prejudice they encounter.

Learning point

Stonewall is a charity using a variety of inventive methods to challenge hetero-assumptive culture and make LGBTQ lifestyles more visible.

Their 'Diversity Champions' programme gives advice to employers and employees on developing good practice regarding sexual orientation. The blue logo, which qualifying businesses are allowed to add to their promotional material, shifts our expectations and brings the issues of LGBTQ rights and equality to the fore in an everyday context.

See www.stonewall.org.uk/at_work/diversity_champions_programme/default
.asp

Their downloadable 'different family' mothers' and fathers' day cards, featuring a variety of families of different genders and ethnicities are free (which may be an important consideration for children, to whom this would be particularly relevant) and might be a creative means of supporting and educating children.

See www.stonewall.org.uk/media/current_releases/5391.asp

Clearly cheap or free services are important in counteracting exclusion, but perhaps particularly so where users may need to conceal their use from others:

Example

A senior practitioner at London Friend described a client who had experienced serious trauma as a result of coming out but had been able to recover quickly as she had a high level of ego strength: 'She was highly educated but had left [her country of origin] because she was threatened with murder and arrived as a refugee. [She] didn't want to go out of her house, so we helped her build a network of support in this country . . . She was able to access the inner resources, which she always had, and apply them to different circumstances. Without that [inner self-belief], the prognosis is not always so good'.

As explored earlier, Cathy was able to use education and access services to support her coming-out and acceptance of her identity in the face of considerable opposition. By contrast, the woman in our next example, Linda, had the added complication of multiple vulnerabilities challenging her attempt to come out.

Linda is an 18-year-old woman diagnosed with mild learning difficulties who is on the autistic spectrum. She was excluded from her FE college following a series of threatening and disruptive outbursts aimed at her tutor, a lesbian who was out to her colleagues but not her students. On her final day at college, she disclosed to her tutor that she 'had feelings for her . . . knew that nothing could happen, but thought she should know'. The tutor contained this disclosure appropriately and researched LGBTQ services for Linda. As Linda needed assistance accessing transport and internet and library services, however, her options were limited. Her tutor was the only 'gay-friendly' person she had encountered; her only regular contact outside college was her mother, who publicly belittled her as 'useless (and) never amounting to anything' and with whom she had a poor relationship.

After leaving college, Linda became more withdrawn and unwilling to leave her house. She was also silent and unresponsive at interviews arranged by Connexions for other colleges, effectively sabotaging them.

Linda already experienced habitual exclusion and ridicule as a person with learning difficulties from various sources, most crucially, her mother. Rather than the potential confiding relationship that might have built her self-esteem, she is rejected. (See Chapter 5 for further discussion of the impact of learning difficulties.)

Linda's tutor provided care, offered positive affirmation of and maintained an LGBTQ-affirmative classroom where homophobia was not tolerated. In this environment Linda felt accepted enough to show how she felt – as someone who was angry and in a lot of pain.

Vulnerable young people may display challenging behaviour with those teachers or other supportive adults whom they have come to trust. They may feel safe enough to display the violent emotion they are battling to contain, particularly if they feel unsupported at home. This frustration can be displaced through seemingly unrelated behaviour, making responding to the underlying need appropriately difficult. This highlights the need for an open-minded approach when assessing the cause of disruptive behaviour and appropriate measures to work with it. It is also vital for staff across different agencies to work together and ensure information is shared effectively and ethically, and is not lost at transition points.

In coming out, Linda advocated something powerful about who she was. Her deeply ingrained experiences of rejection, however, left her so mistrustful of others and of her own worth that she could only disclose this when she was leaving – when there was nothing to gain (her relationship with the tutor was ending) and so had nothing to lose. It is arguable that in the vacuum created at the loss of the source of support for the identity she had chosen, she lapsed into the silence of the identity assigned to her: 'never amounting to anything'.

Learning point

Linda has faced lifelong exclusion prior to coming out, which has compromised her development of ego strength and continues to challenge her independence.

Access to relevant support and social networks, which can be developed without reliance on parents or carers, and can be kept confidential from them, is vital to independence for a vulnerable young person such as Linda.

As illustrated above when faced with multiple vulnerabilities and complicating intersections of concerns over confidentiality, mobility issues, language, culture, and so on, sexuality is often the factor subsumed and sidelined, resulting in a fundamental loss of independence in expressing and experiencing identity. The impact of such sidelining of sexuality issues often remain under-reported diminishing our awareness of the prevalence and extent of such marginalization.

Multiple risk factors

While research is often focused on a single cause of exclusion, such as homophobia or disability, many people experience prejudice and disadvantage in more than one domain. Potential intersections of exclusion are too many to cover exhaustively within the confines of this chapter, but a few examples are provided:

- *Being young LGBTQ and homelessness:*
  - young people are vulnerable to homelessness at a time when they are often discovering their sexuality: 'Research shows that being LGB can be a direct cause of homelessness for young people' (Gold 2005: 8), and brings with it additional vulnerabilities (see Chapter 6);
  - the potential causal factor – their sexuality – may be subsumed in the intervention to assist their homelessness, leaving it unexplored and unassisted and underrepresented.
- *Same-sex domestic violence:*
  - LGBTQ people may be reluctant to disclose their sexuality to professionals, either having experienced or anticipating homophobic prejudice: 'They may not wish to disclose a problem in their relationship because they do not want to "perpetuate the view that same sex relationships are unstable or violent"' (Gold 2005: 21);
  - the lack of awareness of same-sex domestic violence among professionals, the media and wider culture may leave victims unable to name their experience and seek help;
  - there is a lack of appropriate support around domestic abuse, as services are overwhelmingly targeted at heterosexual women and are therefore often unavailable to LGBTQ users, or they may experience homophobia from other service users or staff, leading to reluctance to access a place of safety.
- *LGBTQ and BME:*
  - the potential experience of both racism and homophobia is characterized as '[The] "double jeopardy" associated with being BME

and LGB [which] may increase the likelihood of adverse experiences in mental health care' (Fish 2007: 5);

o services may not reflect the socio-cultural experience of different BME populations, and consequently they may not feel the service is for them and therefore self-exclude;

o services may not be fully accessible, in other words, they may not be offered or advertised in appropriate locations or range of languages;

o research carried out by GALOP (a London-based charity combating LGBT hate crime) and Stonewall indicated that 'Black LGB communities were disproportionately affected by homophobic violence, abuse and harassment' (Sylla and Hodson 2009: 11);

o strong cultural taboos within some communities can leave LGBTQ people feeling that their ethnicity and sexuality are mutually exclusive: 'Being gay can be seen as a denial of ethnicity. For many BME LGB people, their communities are an important support against racism within wider society' (Fish 2007: 6).

Example

A young BME man reported being told by a colleague from another minority ethnic background that 'no one from my country is gay'. The young man was gay but had not disclosed this. He reported feeling extremely anxious around the colleague and began to exhibit symptoms of depression and stress, and added that disclosing his sexuality at work now felt 'out of the question'.

• *LGBTQ and older people:*
  o older people often face desexualization by family, carers – and by sections of the LGBTQ scene – who do not, or prefer not, to consider this element of their identity: 'society behaves as though they no longer have an active sexuality' (Gold 2005: 11). This is a form of exclusion which denies a crucial part of a person's identity. As with internalized homophobia, it can be hugely damaging to self-esteem, and can have mental health implications;

o   older LGBTQ people may face stigma among their contemporaries, which may prove particularly difficult in communal settings such as residential homes or drop-in centres, where there may be little choice of alternative company and may lead to a further sense of isolation.

Learning point

There is a widespread recognition within current literature of the need for greater research into multiple domains of risk, the lack of information on these groups and the potential impact this has on the effectiveness of current interventions.

The Equality and Human Rights Commission's report, *Beyond Tolerance* (2009: 26) argues that the lack of consistent and reliable information nationally on service users' sexual orientation hampers addressing 'the differing needs of lesbians, gay men, bisexual women and bisexual men' and calls for 'monitoring where not already in place'.

In as much as the idea of 'coming out' has penetrated popular media, the image is generally of a single – sometimes cathartic, sometimes traumatic – event, the reality, however, is different. As a man in his mid 30s, in a stable, long-term relationship, who is out to family, friends and work colleagues, Michael found himself unprepared as the recipient of homophobic bullying when he returned to college for vocational training. As Michael said, 'being gay is not necessarily visible . . . in every new job, I have to come out again'. 'It was presumed I was straight – problems began when it emerged I wasn't'.

Michael found himself the victim of direct and indirect homophobic abuse from several fellow students; when he attempted to bring this to the attention of staff, he was told he was 'over-reacting'. Rather than explicitly address the issue and make clear that homophobia was unacceptable in the classroom, thus restoring the boundaries for safe work, nothing was said; instead staff would occasionally defer to him in front of the class, asking if he felt the content of the lesson was 'alright'.

It was incredibly stressful, being identified like that to the rest of the group, as a trouble-maker. It became a self-fulfilling prophesy as those straight people who were supportive [of me] were assumed to be gay by staff and students alike – allowing them to imply that the problem was ours – we needed to change.

Michael found himself isolated and his actions and choices contextualized solely by his sexuality, an experience he was not used to: 'gay is not necessarily my culture – it's not the only thing to define me'. His experience chimes with a London Friend counsellor's explanation of the need for gay affirmative therapy: 'clients can feel their sexuality is accepted and they can work on other issues. It may be for some clients that sexuality as such is not a presenting issue, but they come because they know they're not going to be pathologized for it' (personal communication 2010).

A complicating factor in addressing the bullying Michael experienced was the claim made by several of the perpetrators that this was an expression of their cultural and religious values, and therefore, a right. Staff were unsure of how to respond to the implication that challenging their behaviour was culturally disrespectful and, as a result, did not contain the situation, leaving Michael isolated and the homophobic paradigm unchallenged.

Learning point: hate crimes legislation

There have been several changes and proposed amendments to hate crime legislation, which have been subject to anticipatory distortion in parts of the media, and confusion around competing rights.

Under the Criminal Justice Act (2003), perpetrators of religious and racial hate crimes could be charged with specific offences related to it, whereas homophobic hate crimes could not. Instead the homophobic motivation would be taken into account when sentencing. The Criminal Justice and Immigration Act (2008) extended protection to cover 'hatred against a group of persons defined by reference to sexual orientation' (UK Government Criminal Justice Act (2008), Section 74).

Considered and ongoing diversity training will support staff in holding such a situation with confidence and thoughtfulness, though it remains the exception to the rule, with 90 per cent of school staff saying they 'have not received specific training on how to tackle homophobic bullying' (Hunt and Jensen 2007: 5).

In *Love Thy Neighbour*, Stonewall's 2008 study of attitudes of people of faith to lesbian and gay people, there was cause for some optimism: 'focus group participants all acknowledge that they live in a society where lesbian and gay people do exist. Twenty years ago it's likely that many would have denied knowing anyone who was gay' (Hunt and Valentine 2008: 7). 'Many participants felt the perception that people of faith were openly and resolutely homophobic was often a result of statements made in public by religious leaders, and the fact that alternative views were not put forward' (Hunt and Valentine 2008: 5). Continued dialogue and efforts for community building at every level are needed to combat tension and negative misperceptions on each side.

Michael's experience reminded me of those LGBTQ case studies I have *not* written because of the difficulty of reaching potential interviewees who come from homophobic communities. An LGBTQ member of such a community may find that they need to stay invisible, simultaneously receiving negative feedback about their (hidden) identity, and remaining isolated from potential support; thus the most vulnerable become the least supported.

Learning point

Recent research by London Friend found a profound lack of services for isolated LGBTQ groups, in particular older LGBTQ, disabled LGBTQ and LGBTQ who are not able to come out for cultural reasons. As a result, they have launched a phone line, 'Health at Friend', offering befriending and support to help address this. The lack of services for LGBTQ facing multiple risks of exclusion, however, remains acute, especially outside urban centres.

London Friend highlights the need for greater cross-agency support and communication to work with vulnerable groups. Their relationship with organizations such as The Refugee Council spreads awareness and assists in finding the right referral for a vulnerable client.

Conclusion

Throughout this case study we have seen the particular vulnerability of LGBTQ individuals to having their identity silenced in a culture that assumes heterosexuality as 'the norm'. Challenging that paradigm of normality is crucial to combating the susceptibility to risk of adults in the LGBTQ population. To do this, three strands of visibility need to be addressed:

First, fostering a LGBTQ affirmative culture, in both education and wider culture, provides positive role models for young LGBTQ people, and builds context of acceptance from peers and adults which challenges homophobia.

Second, a high visibility of LGBTQ awareness in all services offered creates an environment in which LGBTQ users may feel more able to consider and disclose their sexuality, and keeps it a real and present consideration for service providers, who may assume heterosexuality, or lose sight of it in addressing other vulnerabilities.

Finally, failure to consistently gather information on LGBTQ presence and needs when collecting data for service provision has been identified by studies such as the Equality and Human Rights Commission's (EHRC) report, *Beyond Tolerance*, as a serious failure in ensuring that adequate and relevant services are available. As the EHRC state: 'there is a vital difference between privacy and invisibility' (2009: 6).

Challenging visibility is essential to combating exclusion, but is of little use without a warm welcome to potential LGBTQ service users. The EHRC's report continues: 'New research for the Commission indicates that homophobia still significantly impacts on the lives of LGB men and women and remains entrenched within institutions and communities' (2009: 5).

For the most excluded members of the LGBTQ community, informed and affirming contact with teachers, medical staff and social or youth workers may be particularly important. Workers in what might be termed the 'caring professions' must be alert to, and challenge, their own prejudices and subconscious cultural assumptions and work to create an open-minded and non-judgemental environment where practitioners may make the most profound impact for good.

Reflection on practice

If we are to challenge the harm caused by vulnerability arising from sexual orientation, practitioners from all sectors of social, medical and educational work need to:

- offer positive affirmation of LGBTQ community to ensure a safe environment for all;
- keep abreast of new developments, legislation, services and organizations that may be relevant to their clients;
- build relationships with projects and agencies and refer clients onto them, as appropriate;
- be mindful of the multiple and complex effects of (potentially undisclosed) homophobic experiences on a client's mental health and well-being.

Using this as a starting point in all practices helps identify the most vulnerable users and deliver interventions in a timely and relevant fashion.

Notes

1   Our expectations must be broadened to allow for multiple identities and greater complexity to combat exclusion. In recognition of this, the case study will use the term 'LGBTQ' to express the other, often excluded in discussions of sexual orientation, with the exception of reporting organizations with specifically narrower remits (i.e. Stonewall, a Lesbian, Gay and Bisexual charity).
2   Personal correspondence, 2009.

References

Bartlett, A., Glenn, S. and King, M. (2009) 'The response of mental health professionals to clients seeking help to change or redirect same-sex orientation' retrieved 15th February 2010 from http://www.biomedcentral.com/1471–244X/9/11.

Dick, S. (2008) Homophobic hate crime. Available at: www.stonewall.org.uk/what_we_do/2583.asp.

Equality and Human Rights Commission (2009) *Beyond Tolerance.* Available at: www.equalityhumanrights.com/fairer-britain/beyond-tolerance-sexual-orientation-project/index.htm.

Fish, J. (2007) *Lesbian, Gay and Bisexual (LGB) People from Black and Minority Ethnic Communities.* Available at: www.dh.gov.uk/publications.

Gold, D. (2005) *Sexual Exclusion: Issues and Best Practices in Lesbian, Bisexual and Gay Housing and Homelessness.* London: Shelter.

Guasp, A. (2007) *The Teachers' Report.* London: Stonewall.

Hunt, R. and Jensen, J. (2007) *The School Report.* Available at: www.stonewall.org.uk/education_for_all/default.asp.

Hunt, R. and Valentine, G. (2008) *Love Thy Neighbour.* London: Stonewall.

Sylla, J. and Hodson, M. (2009) *The Big Update: The Sexual Health Needs of Black Gay Men and Black Men Who Have Sex with Men.* Available at: www.gmfa.org.uk/aboutgmfa/our-work/bigup

Further resources

Stonewall: National Lesbian, Gay and Bisexual charity
www.stonewall.org.uk
Pace: Promoting mental health of LGBT community
www.pacehealth.org.uk
Kenric: National Lesbian social group
www.kenric.org

Bi.org: International Bisexual directory
http://bi.org
UK Black Pride: Celebrating Black LGBT culture
www.ukblackpride.org.uk
UK Black Out: virtual community for black LGBT people
www.ukblackout.com
The Safra Project: working with LGBT women who identify as Muslim either
    culturally or religiously/www.safraproject.org
UK Lesbian and Gay immigration group: Immigration rights for same sex couples
    and asylum seekers
www.uklgig.org.uk
Broken Rainbow: support for and research into same sex domestic violence
www.broken-rainbow.org.uk
London Friend: Promoting wellbeing of LGBT people
www.londonfriend.org.uk
Regard: National organisation of Disabled Lesbians, Gay Men, Bisexuals and
    Transgendered People
www.regard.org.uk
Schools-Out: National organisation for equality in education
www.schools-out.org.uk
Gendered Intelligence: Arts based youth around gender and trans-awareness
    training
www.genderedintelligence.co.uk
The Gender Trust: supporting all affected by gender identity issues
www.gendertrust.org.uk

11 What makes a Gypsy or Traveller vulnerable?

Margaret Greenfields

This case study discusses the diverse ways in which Gypsy and Traveller communities experience multi-factorial social risk – for example in inequality of access to appropriate accommodation; experiences of racism and discrimination; and barriers to accessing health care and education. Gypsies and Travellers have been identified by a range of agencies including the Department of Communities and Local Government and the Equalities and Human Rights Commission (and formerly the Commission for Racial Equality (CRE)) as extremely vulnerable groups across numerous domains, leading to significantly lower life expectancy, economic exclusion, increased rates of morbidity, risk of early criminalization and vulnerability to mental ill-health. The case study will look at life-course vulnerability and examples of good practice in engaging with Gypsy and Traveller community members to enhance their status and access to social care.

Gypsies and Travellers have been recognized as one of the most marginalized, vulnerable and socially excluded populations in Britain today (CRE 2006; Cemlyn et al. 2009). Although members of these communities are in common discourse identified by their preferred accommodation type and nomadic way of life, residence in 'trailers' or leading a highly mobile life is not in fact crucial to their legal and ethnic identity as Gypsies and Travellers. Romany Gypsies (including Welsh Gypsies), Irish Travellers and Scottish Traveller-Gypsies are all in fact recognized in law as ethnic minorities (Clark and Greenfields 2006; Cemlyn et al. 2009), although 'New Travellers'[1] are not a distinct ethnic group and are therefore not protected by the Race Relations Act. Accordingly, for 'ethnic Gypsies and Travellers' it is their cultural and racial characteristics which define them as members of their communities rather than *where* or *how* they live. Estimates of the size of the Gypsy and Traveller population in Britain are problematic in the absence of ethnic monitoring, limited administrative statistics which identify these populations, and their exclusion from census categories.[2] However, at the beginning of the decade it was calculated that there were approximately 300,000 members of these communities in Britain (Morris and Clements 2002). With a high rate of population increase, estimated at 3 per cent per annum (Niner 2003), the community is growing at a rapid rate, akin to some other minority communities (e.g. Bangladeshi) and thus there is an urgency in identifying their needs and ensuring the provision of appropriate services (including access to accommodation) to avoiding these populations' decline into ever-deepening social exclusion and poverty.

Although the most 'visible' members of these community reside in 'traditional' accommodation (caravans/trailers/mobile homes), it is believed that over half of Gypsies and Travellers live in housing (CRE 2006). While considerable evidence exists to demonstrate that the concept and actuality of 'travelling' is inextricably bound up into Gypsy and Traveller identities and culture (Greenfields 2010) common misunderstandings about their legal and ethnic status as minority groups in many cases leads to service providers (as well as members of the public) assuming that someone ceases to be a 'Gypsy' or a 'Traveller' once they live in conventional housing. This misunderstanding (see further below) can be a cause of great distress to populations who are understandably proud of their heritage and history and moreover can lead to problems in accessing services where some agencies are unclear of cultural and practical concerns which can make it difficult for vulnerable members of these populations to engage with mainstream services regardless of where they live.

The Department for Communities and Local Government, the Equalities and Human Rights Commission and the Race Equality Foundation have all recognized the specific risks faced and hardships experienced by Gypsies and Travellers, including those living in housing, resident on 'authorized' sites (with planning permission) and the most marginalized and vulnerable groups who dwell on 'unauthorized' or roadside sites. A concerted policy drive by a number of government departments and agencies in response to the alarming research findings relating to these communities (see below) has begun to make some inroads into the lack of recognition of the vulnerabilities and barriers faced by these populations. However, widespread fiscal retrenchment and the requirements placed on government departments to reduce outgoings since the Spending Revue of Autumn 2010 has created a fundamentally different operational climate, with targeted Gypsy and Traveller projects rapidly being subsumed into more generalized minority ethnic services. As a result, practitioners and the policy community have expressed concerns that these populations are becoming further marginalized, since the May 2010 election of the British Conservative–Liberal Democrat Government.[3]

Regardless of current government policy approaches and the impact of such political changes on both access to sources of funding and the prioritization of particular communities, incontrovertible evidence exists which identifies a number of key areas (considered separately later) as priorities in terms of supporting Gypsies and Travellers, the majority of whom are vulnerable to exclusion purely by dint of their cultural origins and associated life experiences (the 'ethnic penalty'). When other personal characteristics (i.e. gender or age) are then considered in relation to the core domains of exclusion, the impact of such intersectionality creates a greater risk of already vulnerable individuals changing their status to being actively at risk of significant and long-standing (and potentially inter-generational) harm.

This case study will cover:

- accommodation-related risk (see further Chapter 6 for a broader discussion on this topic);
- health;
- education;
- the Criminal Justice System (see further Chapter 7 for a wider discussion);
- employment-related discrimination and racism;
- good practice in addressing Gypsy and Traveller vulnerability.

Learning point

Gypsies and Travellers have been recorded in Britain since at least the late 15th century, typically following occupations related to entertainment, trading, mending of pots and pans ('tinkling' from which the perjorative term 'tinker' comes) and working in farm and agricultural labour. These trades continued as relatively unchanging occupations for members of their communities until the post World War Two modernization of farming and industry and regulation of planning which minimized opportunities to stop for work. The advent of large-scale agricultural farming techniques from the 1990s onwards which utilize large numbers of migrant farm labourers (see further Chapter 12) has also had a significant impact on economic inclusion and employment opportunities for Gypsies and Travellers.

A number of diverse travelling communities are found in Britain with the largest population being Romany Gypsies, who are an ethnic group of Indic origins, many members of which still speak at least some Romani, a language historically but recognizably related to Hindi and Urdu (Kenrick 1993) and who are found predominantly in England and Wales. Irish Travellers, who are indigenous to Ireland and are the main nomadic community in both Northern Ireland and Eire also reside in relatively large numbers in England and Wales (and to a lesser extent in Scotland), having travelled to Britain in fairly large numbers during the 19th century and subsequent post World War Two boom period in building and related industries. Migration backwards and forwards between Ireland and Britain continues to this day. Irish Travellers are numerically the second largest population of travelling people in Britain. Scottish Gypsy-Travellers are a nomadic community indigenous to Scotland, although small groups of Scottish Travellers are sometimes found elsewhere in Britain.

All three of these groups are recognized in law as minority ethnic communities and are thus protected from discrimination by the Race Relations Acts. Although significant cultural variations exist between all three groups, they are all widely recognized by government departments, and health and social care agencies as being 'at risk' or 'vulnerable communities' as a result of the degree of social exclusion and racism they face in their daily lives (Cemlyn et al. 2009).

Accommodation vulnerability

As identified within Maslow's (1943) hierarchy of need, access to secure accommodation is a fundamental requirement, the satisfaction of which then leads individuals to a situation where more complex needs can be met. Accordingly, the lack of appropriate accommodation for Gypsies and Travellers is the key to understanding the numerous inequalities and barriers to accessing public services which are experienced by members of these communities (CRE 2006; Van Cleemput 2008; Cemlyn et al. 2009). Access to accommodation (whether on sites or in housing) is therefore fundamental to enabling Gypsies and Travellers to avail themselves of health, education and other public services which the majority population takes for granted.

Sites

While between half and two-thirds of the Gypsy and Traveller populations of Britain are believed to live in housing (see further below) the remainder, who live in 'traditional' caravan accommodation may be found in a variety of 'types' of sites, with varying degrees of legal (and thus psychological) security. English planning law places considerable constraints on where a caravan can be 'stationed' and a 'Gypsy or Traveller caravan site' occupies a curious legal status from other types of residential or holiday caravan sites, being

- legally only able to accommodate members of those ethnic minority communities and
- as a result of hostility and racism from sedentary populations, applications for planning permission for such sites experiencing considerably greater opposition than other comparable applications for holiday caravan sites, mobile home sites or other forms of planning permission.

Learning point

One in four Gypsies and Travellers living in caravans does not have a legal place on which to park their home. They are thus in law, homeless, often with minimal access to health, social care and education services (Johnson and Willers 2007; Richardson 2007).

Williams (1999) found that over 90 per cent of applications for Gypsy sites are refused at first hearing, often following orchestrated campaigns by aggrieved (settled, non-Gypsy/Traveller) local residents, leading to resultant community tensions.

In 2007 the government-mandated Independent Task Group (in 'the Briscoe Report') calculated that to provide an authorized site for all homeless Gypsies and Travellers in Britain would require one square mile of land. However, largely as a result of political opposition to the provision of 'public' sites (CRE 2006) the estimated annual cost to town halls of repeated eviction and clean-up of unauthorized sites was calculated at £18 million in a 2006 report by the Commission for Racial Equality.

Gypsy and Traveller sites fall into three main types.

- *Public*: sites provided by local authorities or registered social landlords with 'pitches' rented by tenants on a rental equivalent to payment for living in a housing association or council property. Tenants on 'public' sites usually have to provide their own accommodation (caravan), although rental of the concrete 'pitch' where their caravan is parked is typically in the region of £75–90 a week (Clark and Greenfields 2006). Unlike other 'social tenants', Gypsies and Travellers on rented pitches have no rights to security of tenure and can be evicted at extremely short notice. Both the European Court of Human Rights and the House of Lords have said that that amounts to a breach of human rights. The Labour administration prior to the 2010 election had pledged to amend the law to allow them rights similar to other public sector tenants but this had not occurred prior to the change of administration.
- *Private*: sites which are owned by owner-occupiers or a landlord who rents out 'pitches'. Although tenants usually have to provide their own caravan on some rare occasions a landlord may rent out a caravan to them for use on a pitch. The rationale behind residents' provision of their own caravans is that the tenant is thus able to hitch up their home and move away for work or social events and have flexibility over their way of life. In practice, given the acute shortage of pitches, lack of agricultural work where Gypsies and Travellers can park their

caravan while working on the land, and the risk of having nowhere to return to if tenants leave to go travelling, tenants increasingly remain resident on a site for years at a time with only very temporary periods of travel for work in the summer months (Cemlyn et al. 2009).

- *Roadside*: this type of site is by definition 'unauthorized' and typically consists of residents who are unable to obtain access to a 'public' rented site and cannot afford to purchase land (with or without planning permission) to set up a private site. On occasion 'roadsiders' may be groups of Gypsies and Travellers moving between pre-planned work who have access to a site. New Travellers are overwhelmingly resident on 'roadside' sites as they are very rarely able to access authorized sites or (some) may prefer living a highly nomadic way of life. Homeless residents of 'roadside' sites are the most vulnerable members of the Gypsy and Traveller communities and are subject to frequent evictions, with some studies (Greenfields 2009) finding that families reported being moved on or evicted up to 30 times within a six-week period. Thomason (2006) found that only a low number of roadside families experiencing eviction reported being asked about their health or educational needs or personal circumstances before they were moved on. Other hazards for 'roadside families' include traffic danger, fairly regular occurrences of verbal abuse and, on occasion, racist attacks (e.g. bricks thrown through caravan windows) by passers-by or local residents opposed to their stopping within the neighbourhood. 'Roadsiders' in particular are frequently unable to access appropriate health, education and sanitary facilities with predictably negative impacts on population well-being (Cemlyn et al. 2009).

Private sites may be *'authorized'* (with planning permission granted) or *'unauthorized'* (where an owner-occupier or group of families purchase land and move on and set up a site to reside on prior to applying for or obtaining planning permission). Clear evidence exists to support the proposition that families elect to follow this route in anticipation of refusal of planning permission and opposition to their application (Greenfields 2009). Once in residence on a site an applicant has a significantly greater chance that their planning permission application will be granted (particularly if they have children in need of education or family members with unmet health needs who can access medical care from the stable location) than if they apply before moving onto their land.

Example

A researcher who had previously interviewed a Traveller family who were resident on the 'roadside' saw their caravan at a different location some months later and stopped to say hello. While there, she enquired after the health of their four-year-old daughter who was not visible in the caravan. She was told that some weeks earlier the little girl had been knocked down and killed by a passing lorry as her mother was attempting to get the baby out of the car seat after returning from a shopping trip and parking their car in the lay-by on a busy country road where the family were stopped. The little girl had ignored her mother's instruction not to move and had wandered too far out from the car while the baby was being unstrapped. A minute miscalculation on the child's part, even with her mother only a few feet away, proved fatal in such hazardous conditions.

Gypsies and Travellers in housing

While some Gypsy and Traveller families are happily settled into conventional housing and have willingly exchanged the hardships of living a nomadic life, or residing in a caravan on a site, evidence from Gypsy Traveller Accommodation Assessments (GTAAs) undertaken under the Housing Act 2004 supports findings from a number of earlier studies of Gypsies/Travellers in Housing (for a full discussion see Clark and Greenfields 2006 and Chapter 6) and indicates that between half and two-thirds of Gypsies and Travellers in housing moved into such accommodation as a result of inadequate site provision and exhaustion caused by a constant cycle of eviction, or to meet the health or educational needs of family members.

Older Gypsies and Travellers who are no longer able to live in caravans as a result of lack of suitable adaptations or former residence on sites which are hazardous for people with age-related disability are particularly likely to report having to move into housing against their wishes. Where older or disabled people are accommodated in housing away from close family members or have never before lived in 'bricks and mortar' they are particularly vulnerable to social isolation, depression, and problems with debt, for example arising from difficulties in budgeting for regular bills (rather than the purchase of a gas canister for cooking and heating, or high electricity bills resulting from watching television alone instead of socializing with relatives on the site).

For unhappily or 'forcibly' settled Gypsies and Travellers, residence in such types of accommodation has been found to have profoundly negative impacts on well-being, social functioning and mental health (Power 2004; Cemlyn et al. 2009). In particular, isolation from relatives and community structures resulting from enforced movement into housing and repeated experiences of high levels of racism and discrimination from neighbours (Greenfields and Smith 2007) has been found to lead to significant rates of breakdown of housing placement and return to 'roadside' life (Shelter 2007).

Example

Researchers undertaking an Accommodation Assessment interviewed a family living on an 'unauthorized' private site. They had purchased land and moved onto their land prior to obtaining planning permission after their housing placement had broken down. The family had previously lived on a council (public) site which had been closed down and rather than go 'on the roadside' they had accepted a housing association property. On discovering that their new tenants were Romany Gypsies, neighbours had subjected them to a barrage of anonymous abuse including bedroom windows being broken, racist and obscene graffiti spray-painted onto their house, the windows broken on their small 'touring' caravan parked outside the house, their children being physically bullied when walking to and from the house, and dog faeces pushed through their letterbox. The police made a number of efforts to trace the perpetrators but met a wall of silence among local residents. After four months of abuse and limited support from their landlords who thought that 'it would all settle down when they got used to us because we wasn't Gypsies now we was in a house' the family sold most of their possessions to buy a small parcel of land without planning permission after the mother 'was having bad nerves [a breakdown] – *I was too scared to leave the house in case it was burnt out when we wasn't there and scared they'd do something to it when I was there'*.

Health

Although health practitioners working with Gypsies and Travellers had for many years expressed an anecdotal belief that both sited and housed members of the community suffered disproportionately poor health, prior to the 2004 publication of the Department of Health-funded Sheffield University research into the health status of Gypsies and Travellers (Parry et al. 2004) only a handful of studies had set out to methodically analyse health outcomes and prevalence rates of particular conditions among the nomadic population (e.g. Feder et al. 1993; Jenkins 2004). Early reviews had found considerable discrepancies in health status and access to health care among Gypsy and Traveller patients and the surrounding population. However, the Sheffield University project set out to undertake a full review of existing health evidence pertaining to claims of high rates of miscarriage, still-birth, cardio-vascular disease, premature mortality and morbidity, depression and anxiety among the Gypsy and Traveller community.

The implication of the findings from the Sheffield study were sobering, with the research team reporting that even after controlling for socio-economic status and comparing to other marginalized groups, Gypsies and Travellers have worse health than other communities with 38 per cent having a long-term limiting illness, compared with 26 per cent of gender and age-matched comparators from across a range of minority ethnic communities of similar socio-economic status. The research also supported anecdotal evidence relating to premature morbidity, which is believed to be in the region of 12 years lower life expectancy for women and ten years less for Gypsy and Traveller men than is found among other populations. Strikingly, one study in Leeds found that the average life expectancy for Gypsies and Travellers in that city was 50 years of age (Baker and Leeds REC 2005).

Learning point

The Sheffield study (Parry et al. 2004) found that respiratory problems including asthma, bronchitis and chest pain were found more commonly among Gypsies and Travellers than other communities.

A 'conspicuous finding' related to the excess rates of miscarriages, still-births, neonatal deaths and premature death of older children: 17.6 per cent of Gypsy and Traveller mothers had experienced the death of at least one of their children – in some cases related to accidents, or preventable deaths resulting from poor access to health care (such as vaccination against measles) when on the roadside. In comparison, 0.9 per cent of women from the 'mainstream' settled population have experienced such a loss.

Members of these communities also experienced higher rates of diabetes, stroke and cancer. For Gypsies and Travellers, living in a house was associated with long-term illness, poorer health state and high rates of anxiety. Those who rarely travelled were found to have the poorest health of Gypsies and Travellers interviewed.

For nomadic or roadside Gypsies and Travellers considerable difficulties often exist in accessing medical care as many of these community members report that health workers, including GPs and 'front-line' nursing staff, have a poor understanding of their needs, circumstances and culture. Numerous anecdotal reports exist detailing considerable problems in registering with GPs and/or receiving appropriate care from GP practices. As a result, Gypsies and Travellers tend to make greater use of A&E departments for basic health needs than the general population (Matthews 2008). Repeated eviction can also lead to a break in treatment or failure to access screening programmes which could pick up on significant health problems. Frequent transfer between GP practices or attendance at A&E departments of hospitals in times of crisis mean that often there is no continuity of care or note on records that a person has, for example, been experiencing ongoing chest pain or breathing difficulties, meaning that warning signs may be missed.

The widespread literacy problems experienced by Gypsies and Travellers (whether living on the roadside, on sites or in housing) can impact on knowledge of health problems, appropriate use of medication (e.g. sharing of medication between family members has been anecdotally noted to occur fairly frequently) or attending for appointments where letters relating to dates and required pre-examination actions (such as overnight fasting) are sent out to patients. The highly gendered nature of traditional Gypsy and Traveller communities may also lead to women refusing to be examined by a male doctor or failing to disclose 'embarrassing' symptoms.

Example

A middle-aged woman living on the roadside with her family had not been examined for long-standing gynaecological problems as she had been unable to access a female GP when registered as a 'temporary patient' at local surgeries and was too 'shamed' to let a male examine her. Her daughters eventually convinced her to see a woman doctor who practised near to their temporary site. By the time her test results came back the family had been moved on. "If it hadn't been for that woman driving all around asking until she found me I would have been dead – I had to go in and have the emergency operation straight away".

Goward et al. (2006) reported that overall, Gypsy and Traveller communities (whatever type of accommodation they occupied) held low health expectations, normalizing and accepting their poor health status. They therefore tended to make limited use of health care provision and thus increased their risk of contracting avoidable long-term conditions such as diabetes. The concepts of 'self-reliance' and 'staying in control' were reported (Parry et al. 2004) as combining with fatalistic attitudes and an intense fear of death and fear of bereavement loss (Greenfields 2008) to underpin both respondents' health-related behaviours and responses to diagnosis or treatment advice, particularly as patients aged. For many Gypsies and Travellers therefore, avoidance of preventative care or screening programmes leads to a vicious cycle where, by the time a condition is identified, the prognosis is poor; a finding with profound implications for the success of treatment or improving health-related habits (Dion 2008).

Learning point

As part of the Department of Health 'pacesetters' programme a number of initiatives have been targeted at improving Gypsy and Traveller health with the aims of raising awareness of these communities' health needs and circumstances among health care providers, and also advising community members about the range of services available through the NHS. Core aims include ensuring greater access to NHS services and improved GP registration for Gypsies and Travellers and improved record keeping and sharing of health information on individual patients.

A series of projects have been funded across England and Wales – sometimes with the support of local authorities, housing associations or small charitable funders which use community development approaches to work in partnership with Gypsies and Travellers around health and well-being. The most successful approaches involves inter-agency working and the employment and training of peer health advocates and community advisors who can provide advice on particular conditions to members of their own communities and act as supporters for Gypsies and Travellers negotiating access to services.

Education

Literacy- and education-related vulnerability has a fundamental and cross-cutting impact on the life-chances and well-being of both male and female Gypsies and Travellers with the impacts of educational exclusion having negative repercussions throughout the life-cycle.

Although considerable variation obviously exists in individual attainment (with some highly successful professionals and academics openly discussing their Gypsy or Traveller ancestry), by and large the low educational attainment of Gypsies and Travellers as ethnic groups still fully supports the Ofsted statement that 'traveller pupils are still the group most at risk in the education system. They are one Minority Ethnic group which is too often "out of sight and out of mind"' (Ofsted 1999: 11).

In 2003, it was estimated by the Schools Inspectorate that nationally 12,000 Travelling children were not even registered with a school (Ofsted 2003) and that attendance at school of Gypsy and Traveller pupils was only around 75 per cent of the maximum time possible, the worst attendance profile for any ethnic group. A disproportionate numbers of Gypsy and Traveller children are excluded from school at secondary level (Jordan 2001) and even where children have been making extremely good progress at primary school, there is a steep decline in attainment and attendance at school at secondary level, with boys in particular to all intents and purposes often leaving school at the age of 12 (Bhopal and Myers 2008; Cemlyn et al. 2009). While for highly nomadic or insecurely sited families structural barriers exist to accessing education (Save the Children Fund 2001; Cemlyn et al. 2009), similar patterns of non-attendance (although to a lesser extent) are observed among housed Gypsies and Travellers, with research findings indicating that for cultural reasons parents are often highly reluctant for teenagers of the opposite gender to attend school together and that parents particularly fear exposure to alcohol or drugs within a school setting. A mismatch in expectations and agreement over the value of the formal curriculum has also been identified as a significant barrier to remaining in the education system (Jordan 2001; Cemlyn et al. 2009) and there is clear evidence of Gypsy and Traveller pupils experiencing exceptionally high levels of racism and discrimination both from other students and on occasion teachers, which exacerbates the likelihood of parents supporting or encouraging early school leaving (Lloyd and Stead 2001).

Even for those children who do remain within the formal education system, academic outcomes are often poor. In 2007, only 15 per cent of Irish Travellers and 14 per cent of Gypsy/Roma children left school with five or more A*–C grade GCSEs and a further 33 per cent of Irish Travellers and 20 per cent of Gypsy/Roma children failed to obtain any qualifications (DCSF 2007), many of whom were living at unauthorized sites or were members of families whose top priority was seeking a secure place to live, with education a long way down their list of priorities.

In effect, many Gypsies and Travellers experience a cycle of early school leaving (which may lead to functional illiteracy often repeated through generations), with both adults and children experiencing disrupted education arising because of repeated evictions, or work-related movement, or leaving school at a very young age as a result of disillusionment with the school system and lack of peer and family support within a culture which traditionally values practical skills over academic ones (Derrington and Kendall 2004; Bhopal and Myers 2008; Cemlyn et al. 2009).

Learning point

In Scotland, in a 2006 report on the success of educational interventions the Scottish Traveller Education Programme (STEP) reported that 'pupil "mobility" limits regular school attendance, which for Gypsy/Traveller children has resulted in marked academic underachievement, a subsequent reduction in their life chances, access to job opportunities, and reduced likelihood of participating in life-long learning initiatives' (STEP 2006: 6–7). The research found that across Scotland as a whole little coherence existed in terms of practice and knowledge about Scottish Gypsy-Traveller cultures and learning needs, despite many staff devising individual and flexible ways of supporting children and their families in the context of often intermittent access to education.

Many Travellers reported that (inter-generational) experiences of racist bullying at school led families to attempt to hide their children's ethnicity in educational settings. For children who were 'mobile' and thus obviously recognized as 'Travellers' when they entered into a school the risks of bullying were greatly increased. Traveller boys in particular were likely to become involved in conflict and face exclusion from school as a result of defensive responses to racism.

- The report proposed that to best support children in education and enhance relationships between wider family members and schools: schools should provide Gypsy and Traveller pupils with learning resources that do not draw attention to the fact that they are Travellers, *unless the pupil wishes this to be known.*
- Gypsy and Traveller pupils with interrupted learning require interesting resources as their chronological age may be *widely* divergent from their peers' academic stage (e.g. giving a 10-year-old Traveller child reading materials designed for a 5-year-old because of their 'reading age' will tend to act as a disincentive to learning, can be seen as demeaning and can lead to additional taunts and bullying by other children).
- Schools should ensure that teaching and learning for all pupils includes appropriate (positive) references to and images of Gypsy and Traveller communities, past and present, across subject areas (e.g. Traveller children frequently refer to the fact that learning materials automatically assume children live in 'bricks and mortar' (houses or flats) and little reference is made to co-habiting or wide extended family groups or cultural practices which resonate with their experiences).
- Further information on the work of STEP and a range of downloadable resources on Scottish Gypsy-Travellers and educational issues can be found at: www.scottishtravellered.net/

The implications of functional illiteracy are profound, as in an overwhelmingly written culture, accessing services, dealing with bureaucracy and obtaining employment become significant hurdles for individuals who cannot read and write. Fear of racism has anecdotally been identified as a further barrier to disclosing the reasons for a disrupted education and/or seeking adult literacy support (Cemlyn et al. 2009).

As a result of employment and family-related responsibilities, coupled with frequent movement when young, older Gypsies and Travellers are even less likely to be literate than their children or grandchildren who are likely to have had contact with Traveller Educational outreach services when they were growing up.

Lack of literacy also largely precludes access to use of the internet or new technology which in itself can be a significant hurdle to social inclusion and equality of opportunity for Gypsies and Travellers of any age. For highly mobile Travellers, or those on unauthorized sites without access to fixed phone lines, the expense of mobile phone-linked internet service also limits the potential benefits of becoming IT literate.

Example

Voluntary sector agencies report experiences of working with older, newly housed Gypsies and Travellers (and in some cases, individuals who have had to move into housing as a result of their own or a child's disability) who have failed to complete forms pertaining to tenancies, have not been able to apply for housing benefit or who might not have realized that they are in debt in connection with council tax arrears as they have been unable to read letters sent to them and have been too ashamed to ask for help, or did not understand that they needed to attend an appointment with a relevant agency.

The criminal justice system

Although only limited research has been undertaken into Gypsies and Travellers' experiences of law and the criminal justice system (Cemlyn et al. 2009) an emerging body of publications exist to support anecdotal evidence which indicates that Gypsies and Travellers are 'fast tracked' into the criminal justice system, frequently for minor offences, as a result of a combination of insecure accommodation, literacy problems and ways of communicating which are often regarded as insolent or which cause offence and raise communication barriers in relation to engagement with legal and prison service professionals. Once in prison it may remain difficult for Gypsies and Travellers to remain in contact with family members as a result of inability to write letters, limited funds for telephone calls, family movement for work purposes or as a result of being evicted. Advice and support workers report that particularly among men, cultural pride and a tendency to not 'simply do as they are told' means that young Gypsies and Travellers may experience loss of privileges. Racist bullying (or 'pre-emptive' action to avoid expected racism) has also been identified as a source of conflict with both other prisoners and prison service staff given that anti-Traveller prejudice is as common inside as outside prisons. As for any other prisoner, once a conviction has occurred, access to employment and other opportunities becomes severely minimized. Illiterate Gypsies and Travellers are also unable to avail themselves of educational opportunities while in custody or earn remission from their sentences as a result of their lack of reading and writing skills as attendance at courses is often regarded as a prerequisite to demonstrate rehabilitation.

Example

An advice worker who was interviewed for a research study reported that a young man with no previous convictions (and a pregnant wife) had been arrested on a minor driving offence. He was unable to produce 'his papers' [insurance certificate and driving licence] as they were in a caravan which had been taken to Ireland by a family member who was not expected back in the UK for at least a month. The man who had taken the caravan abroad had then gone to Germany to collect a newly bought car and was not available to find the papers and send on copies or originals to the police station/court. Some question existed as to whether the young man even had a driving licence as he was unable to read and may not have taken his driving test because of the written element of the test. The young man was remanded in custody at a London prison with a reputation for being 'tough' because he was unable to provide an address for bail which was regarded as 'secure' as his family were living on an unauthorized site. His cousin had committed suicide in the same prison 18 months earlier after becoming substance addicted and severely depressed while in prison.

The young man was convicted and sentenced to a period in custody as he was seen as being at risk of absconding. While in prison, problems occurred over receiving family visits as his illiteracy, lack of knowledge of current addresses (given their mobility) and precise dates of birth of family members and their lack of suitable identifying documents meant that 'visiting order' forms could not be completed correctly. Extreme cultural isolation in prison, claustrophobia and racist bullying led to a serious suicide attempt within two weeks of being convicted.

Employment-related discrimination and racism

Although many Gypsies and Travellers follow 'traditional' self-employment patterns and work in family groups in gardening, building works and trading (e.g. in cars imported from the continent or selling carpets at markets), there are reports of growing unemployment and welfare dependency for members of these communities (Cemlyn et al. 2009). The recent economic recession is likely to have impacted particularly severely on Gypsies and Travellers as a result of often limited educational qualifications which may diminish opportunities for seeking alternative employment or training if primary (traditional) income sources are depleted (CRE 2006).

Niner's (2003) study on behalf of the government reported that 'on seven out of ten [public] sites a minority of households work', with over one-third of site managers noting that less than 10 per cent of residents were in employment. Given that the network of approximately 320 local authority sites accommodates roughly one-third of the caravan-dwelling Gypsy and Traveller community (Communities and Local Government (CLG) 2009) economic exclusion rates could thus be extremely high and rising. Given emerging evidence (Cemlyn et al. 2009) that relatively high rates of disability (or acting as a carer for a disabled person) are found among Gypsy and Traveller research respondents, policy shifts and expectations pertaining to the employment and training responsibilities of individuals with a diverse range of disabilities are therefore likely to impact particularly hard on this section of their community through increased pressure to engage with paid employment, although literacy and technical (e.g. IT) skills are likely to be lacking, which in practice may have the effect of compounding their exclusion from employment.

Traditionally accommodated Gypsies and Travellers (resident in caravans) also refer to the difficulties facing them in seeking and retaining employment once they are known to live at a caravan site (Greenfields and Smith 2009), with many potential employers discriminating against applicants on the basis of their address alone.

For Gypsies and Travellers who are employed, despite theoretical protection from discrimination arising from their membership of an ethnic group, considerable evidence exists to demonstrate that members of these communities seek to hide their ethnicity from workmates to avoid racism or workplace bullying (Greenfields 2008; Cemlyn et al. 2009).

Example

A young woman who lived on a 'public site' worked for six months in a local jewellers' shop, having given a housed friend's address when she applied for the job. Her work had been satisfactory and everybody seemed happy with her attendance and performance, to the extent that she was allowed to count the jewelry in and out of the safe while her colleagues were working in other sections of the shop or filling or emptying display cases. Once it was known that she was a Gypsy she was no longer left alone with the gold and she heard 'comments' made about Gypsies stealing and their liking for gold. She left her post shortly afterwards. This clear case of constructive dismissal was not followed up by the young woman as she was too humiliated by the situation and in any event probably unaware of her legal rights.

Overall, experiences of casual racism and discrimination in employment, education and a range of other settings (e.g. being refused access to pubs, launderettes and leisure centres) are reported by over 90 per cent of Gypsies and Travellers who have participated in Accommodation Assessments which include questions on access to a range of other services. Respondents from across a broad spread of age ranges report that, as a secondary effect of their negative experiences, they are less inclined to engage with other communities and tend to expect hostile reactions from those with whom they come into contact.

Thus the impact of life-long experiences of such discrimination are profound, leading in many cases to a generalized mistrust of 'others' and a tendency to 'hide' ethnicity in social circumstances when not with other Gypsies and Travellers. Hostile newspaper articles and media-driven negative discourse around members of these communities also have an intensely negative effect on community cohesion and in many cases create a vicious cycle of mistrust and lack of communication between Gypsies and Travellers and 'settled' surrounding populations (Richardson 2006).

Good practice in addressing Gypsy and Traveller vulnerability

In order to meet the needs of Gypsies and Travellers who are at risk across a wide variety of domains it is important to work in a sustainable and 'joined-up' way, with agencies being aware of the variety of support needs which can face community members. Awareness of the cross-cutting issues (e.g. literacy, access to accommodation, experiences of racism) which increase the risk of members of these communities being at risk of harm should always be taken into account when working with, planning services for, and undertaking community development with Gypsies and Travellers.

In a number of localities, following on from accommodation assessments inter-agency fora have been set up to continue to work with Gypsy and Traveller residents, building upon the networks and trust which have developed while undertaking accommodation need surveys.

It is therefore advisable (where no such fora exist) to explore the potential for inter-agency working to design and deliver coherent services for local (and visiting) Gypsy and Traveller community members. Such holistic working can avoid expensive duplication of resources as well as ensuring that service users are not directed to a number of different agencies who may only have limited knowledge on one element of the concerns which face them. Being sent from 'pillar to post' increases the sense of frustration of many Gypsies and Travellers and can feed the belief that they are a 'forgotten minority'. In contrast, access to an agency or individual who is aware of what may be a variety of very complex needs facing a family can lead to rapid prioritization and delivery of appropriate support services which avoid the risk of deepening social exclusion.

Example

It is critically important to actively consult with and involve members of Gypsy and Traveller communities in the development of local initiatives and materials, as respondents often speak about 'being fed up with having things done "to" us and nobody actually asking us what WE want'. Increased recognition of the importance of community development approaches to working in partnership with Gypsies and Travellers and the growing number of trained and experienced community activists (in some cases employed as outreach workers by local authorities or voluntary sector agencies such as Irish Traveller Movement Britain and Friends, Families and Travellers: see under further reading) means that local community members can often be recruited onto steering groups to assist in devising strategies and providing culturally specific advice on how best to engage with local Gypsies and Travellers.

When designing materials and information sources for community members, it is important that these are written in accessible language and where possible made available in audio format or with graphics and images to ensure that they are suitable for service users who may in some cases have limited literacy skills and who may be too embarrassed or worried about racism to ask someone else to read the leaflets for them. However, be aware that it is demeaning to members of these communities to automatically assume that everyone is unable to read or is living 'on the roadside' – accordingly, sensitive awareness of the issues which may face some Gypsies and Travellers and tailored cultural awareness training for all front-line staff can be an effective way of engaging with myths and confusions about supporting members of these populations.

Learning point

To enable delivery of good quality services ensure that your working environment has resource lists and information on national and local sources of Gypsy and Traveller advice, for example Traveller Education Services, local voluntary sector agencies working with members of these communities or specialist health workers. Establish links with agencies who may be able to help or act as advocates when you are supporting Gypsy and Traveller service users.

Challenge negative stereotyping of Gypsy and Traveller communities heard in both employment and social contexts and suggest that people take the time to find out more about the lifestyles and needs of members of these communities.

See further the ground-breaking 'Gypsies and Travellers Myth-busting' booklet produced by Bristol County Council, which discusses Gypsy and Traveller culture, legal status, social exclusion issues, good practice in community engagement and lists sources of local advice and support.

http://www.bristol.gov.uk/ccm/content/Community-Living/Equality-Diversity/files/information/gypsies-and-travellers-mythbusting-booklet.en

---

Conclusion

As has been demonstrated with reference to a number of areas, Gypsies and Travellers are communities who are 'at risk' across the life-course – with significantly less likelihood of being safely born, reaching adulthood, achieving an age which is commensurate with the life-expectancy of surrounding populations and, additionally, being more likely than mainstream (and even other minority ethnic) communities to suffer poor health, disability and poverty arising from social and financial exclusion.

In addition, there are strongly gendered dimensions of social exclusion and inequalities experienced by Gypsies and Travellers as women tend to report greater levels of contact with bureaucracy than do men – partially as a result of their generally higher literacy levels and partly due to cultural expectations that paid work is within the male realm and dealing with education, local authority and health personnel are part of a woman's role. In addition, for 'ethnic' Gypsies and Travellers, home and domestic responsibilities are firmly the responsibility of women and the necessity of keeping an ordered home amid the complexities of frequent movement and in the face of widespread hostility and racism, can for many women lead to high levels of anxiety and stress. Additionally, 'newly housed' women often report that the combination of dealing with interactions with neighbours who are frequently lacking in knowledge of Gypsy and Traveller culture and who may be hostile to their new neighbours, isolation from close extended family with whom women have often lived since birth, financial and budgeting difficulties, literacy problems and making the transition to a new form of accommodation, can prove overwhelming and lead to additional domestic pressures, particularly when men are away working with relatives, and household responsibilities fall completely onto the shoulders of women (see further Cemlyn et al. 2009).

In the light of the above it is therefore argued that, by definition, Gypsies and Travellers are at risk of vulnerability and should by virtue of their membership of a class of people be accorded the opportunity to access staff with specialist knowledge of their circumstances and if appropriate tailored support to mitigate the impacts of centuries of exclusion.

Notes

1   'New Travellers' are a non-ethnic nomadic group which emerged from the itinerant festival goers of the 1970s–1980s who travelled together and resided in converted vehicles or in some cases horse-drawn caravans. Many 'New Travellers' consciously adopted a 'green' way of life and took on practices which to some extent were being abandoned by ethnic Gypsies and Travellers in the post-modern world. Although minority ethnic Travelling peoples with centuries of history tend to be scathing of the 'authenticity' of New Travellers who are often described as 'hippies' or 'middle-class imposters', members of this community have a distinct and emerging culture and practice of their own and we are now seeing third-generation 'New' Travellers who have grown up 'on the road' and face similar educational, employment and health barriers and concerns to that of 'traditional' Gypsies and Travellers.

2   For the first time the 2011 Census categories will include the option of Romany Gypsy or Irish Traveller. This will greatly assist in identifying numbers of these minority communities with the UK. Unfortunately the proposed abolition of the National Census from 2021 (Gourlay 2010) means that no coherent administrative data set pertaining to Gypsies and Travellers will be developed in future years.

3   See further Threats to Gypsy and Traveller Rights, Guardian Letters Page, available at www.guardian.co.uk/society/2010/jun/04/equality-liberal-conservative-coalition

References

Baker, M. and Leeds REC (2005) *Gypsies and Travellers: Leeds Baseline Census 2004–2005.* Leeds: Leeds REC.

Bhopal, K. and Myers, M. (2008) *Insiders, Outsiders and Others: Gypsies and Identities.* Hatfield: University of Hertfordshire Press.

Cemlyn, S., Greenfields, M., Burnett, S., Matthews, Z. and Whitwell, C. (2009) *Review of Inequalities Experienced by Gypsy and Traveller Communities.* London: Equalities and Human Rights Commission (EHRC).

Clark, C. and Greenfields, M. (eds) (2006) *Here to Stay: The Gypsies and Travellers of Britain.* Hatfield: University of Hertfordshire Press.

Commission for Racial Equality (CRE) (2006) *Common Ground: Equality, Good Race Relations and Sites for Gypsies and Irish Travellers: Report of a CRE Inquiry in England and Wales.* London: CRE.

Communities and Local Government (CLG) (2009) *Biannual Gypsy and Traveller Caravan Count – July 2009.* London: CLG.

Department for Children, Schools and Families (DCSF) (2007) *National Curriculum Assessment, GCSE and Equivalent Attainment and Post–16 Attainment by Pupil Characteristics, in England 2006/07.* London: DCSF.

Derrington, C. and Kendall, S. (2004) *Gypsy Traveller Students in Secondary Schools.* Stoke on Trent: Trentham Books.

Dion, X. (2008) Gypsies and Travellers: cultural influences on health. *Community Practitioner*, 81(6): 31–4.

Feder, G., Vaclavik, T. and Streetly, A. (1993) Traveller Gypsies and childhood immunisation: a study in East London. *British Journal of General Practice*, 43: 281–4.

Gourlay, C. (2010) Witches and Jedis put hex on UK census. *The Times*, 14 February.

Goward, P., Repper, J., Appleton, L. and Hagan, T. (2006) Crossing boundaries: identifying and meeting the mental health needs of Gypsies and Travellers. *Journal of Mental Health.* 15(3): 315–27.

Greenfields, M. (2008) *'A Good Job for a Traveller?': Exploring Gypsies and Travellers' Perceptions of Health and Social Care Careers.* High Wycombe. Buckinghamshire New University/Aimhigher South East.

Greenfields, M. (2009) *Gypsies, Travellers and Accommodation, Better Housing Briefing 10: A Race Equality Foundation Briefing Paper.* London: Race Equality Foundation.

Greenfields, M. (2010) Romany Roots: Gypsies and Travellers in Britain, sustaining belonging and identity over 600 years of nomadising. In L. De Pretto, G. Macri and C. Wong (eds) *Diasporas: Revisiting and Discovering* (e-book).

Greenfields, M. and Smith, D. (2007) Travellers and housing: social housing exchange and the construction of communities. Unpublished conference paper, Social Policy Association Conference, July 2007, Birmingham.

Greenfields, M. and Smith, D. (2009) Turning a penny a new way: economic strategies of housed Gypsies and Travellers. Unpublished conference paper Social Policy Association Annual Conference, University of Edinburgh 29 June–2 July.

Independent Task Group (2007) *The Road Ahead: The Final Report to Ministers of the Independent Task Group on Site Provision and Enforcement.* Available at http://www.communities.gov.uk/documents/housing/pdf/roadahead.pdf.

Jenkins, M. (2004) *No Travellers! A Report of Gypsy and Traveller Women's Experiences of Maternity Care.* London: Maternity Alliance.

Johnson, C. and Willers, M. (2007) *Gypsy and Traveller Law.* London: LAG.

Jordan, E. (2001) Exclusion of Travellers in state schools. *Educational Research,* 43(2): 117–32.

Karlssen, S. (2007) *Better Health Briefing Three Ethnic Inequalities in Health: The Impact of Rracism.* London: Race Equality Foundation.

Kenrick, D. (1993) *Gypsies from India to the Mediterranean.* Toulouse: CRDP Midi Pyrénées.

Lloyd, G. and Stead, J. (2001) 'The boys and girls not calling me names, and the teachers to believe me': name calling and the experiences of Travellers in school. *Children and Society,* 15: 361–74.

Maslow, A. (1943) A theory of human motivation. *Psychological Review,* 50(4): 370–96.

Matthews, Z. (2008) *The Health of Gypsies and Travellers in the UK.* London: Race Equality Foundation.

Morris, R. and Clements, L. (2002) *At What Cost? The Economics of Gypsy and Traveller Encampments.* Bristol: Policy Press.

Niner, P. (2003) *Local Authority Gypsy/Traveller Sites in England.* London: Office of the Deputy Prime Minister.

Ofsted (1999) *Raising the Attainment of Minority Ethnic Pupils.* London: Ofsted.

Ofsted (2003) *Provision and Support for Traveller Pupils.* London: Ofsted.

Parry, G. et al. (2004) *The Health Status of Gypsies and Travellers in England.* Sheffield: ScHARR.

Power, C. (2004) *Room to Roam: England's Irish Travellers.* London: Brent Irish Advisory Service.

Richardson, J. (2006) *The Gypsy Debate: Can Discourse Control?* Exeter: Imprint Academic.

Richardson, J. (2007) *Providing Gypsy and Traveller Sites: Contentious Spaces.* York: Chartered Institute of Housing/Joseph Rowntree Foundation.

Save the Children Fund (2001) *Denied a Future? The Right to Education of Roma/Gypsy & Traveller Children in Europe (Vol 2: Western and Central Europe).* London: SCF.

Shelter (2007) *Good Practice Briefing: Working with Housed Gypsies and Travellers.* London: Shelter.

STEP (2006) *Impact of National Guidance: Inclusive Educational Approaches for Gypsies and Travellers within the Context of Interrupted Learning, Schools and Practice.* Edinburgh: STEP.

Thomason, C. (2006) *Here to Stay: An Exploratory Study into the Needs and Preferences of Gypsy/Traveller Communities in Cheshire, Halton and Warrington.* Chester: Cheshire, Halton & Warrington Race Equality Council.
Van Cleemput, P. (2008) Health impact of gypsy sites policy in the UK. *Social Policy & Society*, 7(1): 103–17.
Williams, T. (1999) *Private Gypsy Site Provision.* Harlow: Advisory Council for the Education of Romany and other Travellers (ACERT).

Further resources

Equalities and Human Rights Commission (EHRC), available at: www.equality humanrights.com/en/publicationsandresources/Pages/InequalitiesGypsyand Traveller.aspx
Friends, Families and Travellers (FFT) is the only national charity for Gypsies and Travellers to engage with all types and communities of Travellers (Romany Gypsies, Irish Travellers, Scottish Gypsy-Travellers and New Travellers). In addition to their referral service, advice and policy units which monitors and engages with accommodation issues this organization has a thriving Health project. Recent FFT web-publications and a range of links to organizations and journal articles on Gypsy and Traveller communities can be accessed from their website www.gypsy-traveller.org/).
Irish Traveller Movement (Britain) works predominantly with members of the Irish Traveller community across the UK. They are the British branch of an international lobbying and policy organization aimed at improving the situation of Irish Travellers in Europe. ITMB are also actively engaged in health and community development activities. A range of articles and resources are available from their website at: www.irishtraveller.org.uk/. Each Autumn ITMB hosts a well-attended policy conference which deals with issues relevant to all 'ethnic' Gypsy and Traveller communities, for example criminal justice, accommodation, health etc.

12 Vulnerable adult migrants in East Anglia

David Bailey

This case study begins by outlining the key issues faced by migrant workers to the UK and discusses the role of local authorities in working with service providers who engage with such potentially vulnerable workers. In the remainder of the chapter a case study based on the author's own locality is used to discuss experiences, risk factors and indicators of vulnerability within the employment sector for migrant adults. Particular attention is paid to the impacts on health and well-being and risk of exploitation arising from low pay, illegal/unfair deductions from pay, unsafe workplaces, limited rights to leave (including maternity leave), insecurity at work and related issues.

Despite the 21st-century media preoccupation with refugees, asylum seekers and migrant workers entering the country, the history of migration to the United Kingdom is by no means new, stretching back thousands of years (Winder 2005). Whether to escape persecution or to improve their personal circumstances, time and again new arrivals from Europe, the Commonwealth and further afield have come to Britain, bringing their skills, knowledge and expertise.

But along with those who have 'transferable and desirable' skills which meet the current identified needs of the economy, are those who move for economic reasons to give themselves and their families opportunities which are closed to them in their own countries. In certain instances (particularly for those moving to low-skilled or precarious employment) migration can lead to exploitation of those who are vulnerable to risk, or have been misled over the circumstances awaiting them (Jayaweera and Anderson 2009). For all such migrants, a potential exists that their vulnerability can lead to abuse (Craig et al. 2007).

Learning point

There is no universally agreed definition of the term 'migrant worker' with different agencies, bodies and governments using their own slightly different definitions. The definition employed by the Department of Work and Pensions, (Robinson 2002) characterized migrants as 'those recently arrived overseas workers who have arrived in the UK' or those who have 'applied for a national insurance number within the previous year'. Inevitably, such a broad definition embraces a range of situations and circumstances which depend upon the duration of stay, validating mechanisms involved when entering Britain and the formal employment status of the migrant. While highly skilled medical or business professionals are thus just as much 'migrant workers' as low-paid casual farm labourers or people working in the catering trade, within this case study the focus is on migrant workers who are not protected from vulnerability and risk of exploitation by virtue of their ability to access well-regulated international employment procedures or as a result of being members of a profession.

The UK has seen a significant rise in the number of migrant workers since 2004 when the European Union expanded to include the 'Accession States' (the A8) comprising the following countries: Czech Republic, Estonia, Hungary, Latvia, Lithuania, Poland, Slovakia, Bulgaria and Romania. Increased globalization and the availability of low-cost air fares have also encouraged foreign nationals to exploit the higher quality of life and employment opportunities in the UK. While many A8 migrants are highly skilled and literate in several languages, many such workers are employed in low-skilled, relatively casualized employment such as catering, hotel, factory or farm labour sectors (Glossop and Shaheen 2009).

This inward migration has impacted on both cities and rural areas across the United Kingdom in a way which has rarely occurred so uniformly in relation to earlier waves of migration, which have often focused on particular industries (e.g. clothing factories in the 1950s) or localities (such as London or the Midlands). A8 migrants are found in all countries of Britain, including areas such as rural Wales and Scotland (DWP 2006; Scottish Association of Citizens Advice Bureaux (SACAB) 2006) where local residents and professionals who will come into contact with new migrants may have only had limited knowledge of, or contact and experience with, interacting with people of other cultures and nationalities. Thus while migrant populations are frequently perceived to be an urban phenomenon, in reality, in the past few years, they may also be found in large numbers in rural areas, making a huge contribution to the local economy, and often undertaking work where there is no suitable or insufficient labour force.

This geographic spread of new migrants, coupled with the scale of migration and the demographic profile of these workers – mainly young adults without dependants – has however had significant implications for local authorities and their communities. In particular, in order to attempt to map the changing needs of their residents, local authorities have been required to explore new ways to:

- improve data and intelligence about migration to the area and the impacts of demographic change when developing strategies and plans;
- build new partnerships with migrants' employers and the voluntary and statutory sector engaging with new migrants to understand particular concerns and adapt services to meet the needs of a changing population;
- provide information to new migrants about living and working in the UK;
- ensure the housing of migrants meets proper standards through regulating housing in multiple occupation and promoting community cohesion by working with both new and existing communities.

The relative invisibility of many migrant workers, the potential for language barriers to exist, workers' limited knowledge of their rights, and the lack of public debate about their needs, means however that despite the best efforts of local authorities and service providers, where risk of exploitation exists, agencies and front line staff may not be aware of how to engage effectively with migrant workers to ensure that potentially vulnerable adults do not become subject to abuse. In the remainder of this chapter, a case study format is utilized to illustrate risk factors faced by migrant workers in a rural area and to demonstrate ways of responding to the concerns identified by front line staff who come into contact with potentially vulnerable workers.

Learning point

The employment of migrant workers in rural areas of the UK is not a new practice. The use of Gypsies, Irish harvest migrants as well as the employment of 'navvies' to construct the nation's infrastructure in the 19th and 20th centuries are a few illustrations of the historic use of migrant workers in driving and strengthening the economy (Winder 2005).

The case study location

Cambridgeshire in Eastern England is a good example of an area which combines both urban and rural areas. The country has two cites, Cambridge (a long-established university city which is used to inward migration from students over many centuries), and the expanding city of Peterborough, where over 120 different languages are spoken (internal local authority statistics). However, the vast majority of the county is a rural hinterland which, until the arrival of the migrant population in recent years, had not experienced high levels of inward migration.

The District of Fenland, lying to the east of Peterborough and north of Cambridge, is one of five districts in the county. Fenland has four market towns within its boundaries and one of the highest levels of multiple index deprivation in the county. The mid census population estimate for the District of Fenland calculates that there are 91,300 people living in the district.

Fenland District shares boundaries with a number of other local authorities, including the District of South Holland in Lincolnshire, the District of West Norfolk (in Norfolk), and the county of Huntingdonshire, as well as Peterborough, King's Lynn and East Cambridgeshire. Thus effective inter-agency working and planning often requires liaison with other local authority areas. Out of the adjoining districts, Fenland in particular has seen an influx of foreign nationals, attracted by the prospect of seasonal agricultural labour. Since 2005, it is estimated that over 9000 Eastern Europeans have lived and/or worked in Fenland (anecdotal evidence and internal local authority data). The highest numbers of migrants have settled in the vicinity of Wisbech, a town whose industry is predominately based around agriculture and food processing. Even if initially attracted to the locality to access seasonal work, A8 migrants are increasingly remaining in Fenland after seasonal work has ended, taking up employment in the manufacturing and service industries.

To understand the impact of inward migration on this scale, and to identify the issues faced by the migrant population, in 2009 the Council and its partners commissioned research to identify the situation in the district and plan future services to meet needs. The findings from this study heightened awareness of the risks faced by this population, identifying both 'obvious' and multi-faceted hidden vulnerabilities. A key finding from the study was that the issues faced by migrant workers and their families within a rural location seldom exist in isolation, for example, where employment exploitation, accommodation problems and language concerns all co-exist, these can coalesce to push an individual into crisis which in turn may (for example) lead to conflict with the legal system through misunderstanding of regulations or where someone takes a calculated risk in response to a desperate situation. Problems and vulnerabilities experienced by migrant workers are therefore frequently inter-related and often form part of a wider, more complex set of factors. For that reason, it is sometimes difficult to distinguish between a discrete, free-standing problem and one which is a symptom of a wider set of variable factors, a situation which can create difficulties for front line staff seeking to work with a migrant worker client facing a complex web of concerns.

The research findings

The study found that the main risk factors and areas of life where migrant workers are most vulnerable fall into the following categories: employment-related problems, accommodation issues, linguistic and education concerns, legal/policing contacts, health and social security difficulties. When any one area is affected, it would appear particularly easy for migrant workers to become vulnerable across a further domain (e.g. loss of accommodation resulting from health problems). Workers who were already potentially at risk as a result of a personal characteristic (e.g. gender, age or disability) were found in some circumstances to be particularly vulnerable to exploitation, thus being pushed into a negative downward spiral. In particular where individuals lacked access to networks and hence had low social capital, they often failed to obtain support which could have mitigated their circumstances. Thus a series of risk factors could intersect to place them at greater risk than other workers who did not possess their particular set of vulnerabilities. Accordingly, responsive planning (and individual support) offered to migrant workers needs to take account of both personal circumstances and the individual's position as a member of a class of migrant workers.

Learning point

Many legal (as well as undocumented) migrants seeking work are vulnerable to exploitation by landlords, employers and by unscrupulous people offering credit and money lending at exorbitant rates of interest. Moreover, in some long-established communities with little experience of migration there may be sensitivity to the settlement of people with different cultural practices. Migrants can therefore face discrimination and racial harassment and find it difficult to report their experiences to the authorities. The children of migrant families may also find it difficult to learn effectively at local schools as they can feel isolated and have problems in making progress through the national curriculum, particularly if language barriers exist. The recent economic downturn and the rise of far Right political parties and an often migrant-hostile media have exacerbated some of these issues further as competition for jobs increases in areas with little available employment.

Employment

Given that the driver for relocation to Britain is access to work for members of migrant communities, it is perhaps inevitable that employment and related issues should feature prominently on the agenda as a key cause of vulnerability for these populations. The research found that participants faced a number of difficulties in the labour market, including problems with specialist migrant employment agencies and 'gang-masters'[1] such as:

- inaccurate representation of the nature of jobs available to the migrant worker, levels of pay, and holiday entitlements;
- inadequate information provided on matters such as their employment and welfare rights and entitlements;
- a lack of transparency and proportionality surrounding the deductions made by the agency from earned income to cover costs of housing, transport and administration;
- failure to honour commitments on matters such as skills development and training.

Example

A local Citizens Advice Bureau reported the case of a man who had worked for several months for his employer before he had an accident at work and broke his arm. His employer told him that he was not entitled to Statutory Sick Pay, even though the legislation confirmed that he was entitled to receive such payment. When he challenged his employer, he was dismissed without notice or payment in lieu of notice.

Housing

The initial impact of migrant families on local housing supply and demand is cushioned by the fact that agencies and employers often arrange accommodation for people whom they have brought to the UK for work or whom they have employed locally. For example, migrants working in the hospitality industry sometimes live in hotel annexes and seasonal agricultural workers are usually accommodated in caravans and converted farm buildings.

Despite the apparent convenience of these arrangements these situations pose challenges for workers and support agencies working with them as the provision of 'tied' housing can result in them being placed in substandard or even illegal provision (e.g unlicensed or dangerously overcrowded accommodation with inadequate sanitary or fire safety provision). Housing issues predominate on the list of problems experienced by migrants.

Particular issues associated with 'tied' housing include.

- loss of a job resulting in loss of accommodation which results in homelessness;
- lack of continuous employment leading to rent arrears and debt to the employing agency;
- accommodation provided is often poor quality, sub-standard and overcrowded;
- sexual harassment experienced by home female migrants in shared/ over-crowded accommodation (International Labour Organization 2009);
- absence of tenancy agreements, undermining security of tenure for migrants;
- accommodation being particularly inappropriate for the needs of families;
- rent levels being often far higher than the equivalent rental charged in the private rented sector.

Local data show that the median pay of migrant workers has been found to be under half that of the wider population (in an area which is already noted as having lower wage levels than anywhere else in Cambridgeshire, and salaries consistently below the UK average), meaning that migrants are often forced to stay in sub-standard accommodation tied to employment or in low-cost, sub-standard private sector housing. The influx of migrant workers, particularly from the Eastern European accession countries, has provided opportunities for exploitation, particularly by unlicensed landlords (McKay and Winkelmann-Gleed 2005).

Issues associated with moving to or living in rented accommodation are:

- the need for a deposit and the payment of rent in advance can be very difficult for low-paid workers;
- affordability, especially in relation to eligibility for Housing Benefits or limits imposed on Housing Benefits for recent migrants;
- insecurity of tenure;
- quality and standard of housing made available to migrants may be lower than that available to other communities.

Houses in Multiple Occupation (HMOs)

These are one of the most visible features of the presence of the A8 migrant population in the Fenland area, and also form one of the main 'flashpoints' with the local population who often resent the presence of intensively occupied premises with frequent movement of (predominantly young, male) residents in and out of the properties located in residential housing areas. Regardless of these concerns, there are often causes for concern regarding the over-occupation and crowding within such housing, with HMOs representing the most 'obvious' symbols of marginalization and exploitation of the new migrant population. The accommodation-related exploitation often has a knock-on effect for neighbours who complain about noise, rubbish and other environmental impacts, which in turn stretches existing capacity within the Council's housing and environmental health services when enquiries and investigations are undertaken.

Homelessness

In the current economic situation the risk of migrants losing jobs is increasing. In turn this has an impact on homelessness rates among Eastern Europeans as sudden unemployment (frequently due to loss of tied accommodation) leads to friction and unrest in the wider community. Given the low wages commonly found among this group and (as is extremely common) lack of savings, coupled with limited English language skills, loss of work among this group leads very quickly to destitution. Not only does street homelessness impact on the wider community but the vulnerability of migrants in these circumstances leads to a high risk of exploitation, particularly for women who may be at risk of being lured into the sex industry as a way out of poverty, or when seeking accommodation with a 'friendly' man (Craig et al. 2007). The risk to all migrants at the cusp of homelessness is evidenced by a number of local cases of assault on rough-sleeping Eastern European migrants (Milmo 2007).

Education and access to information

As many A8 workers come with a basic or excellent command of the English language (and some are conversant in several languages), not all migrants will need access to language training. However, those who are unable to speak English face significant barriers in relation to obtaining employment other than through migrant worker agencies or gangmasters, accessing services and integrating within local communities. They are also those most at risk of exploitation as a result of limited knowledge of their rights (Craig et al. 2007).

Where a migrant worker is unfamiliar with the procedures required on entering the UK they can become lost in a maze of bureaucracy and overly dependent upon their employer who may in some cases exploit them by providing wrong information or allowing them to fall into debt to the agency, for example by telling them they cannot access Housing Benefit or would have to leave the country if they stopped working for a particular gangmaster.

In addition to adult education needs of migrant workers, an increasing number of young families are bringing school-age dependants with them who may either need additional help and support at school to integrate, or have to face racist bullying in educational settings. In some cases, inappropriately, young people and children find themselves acting as translators for their parents and other adults whose English skills are not as developed as their own.

Benefits and entitlements

Work permit holders and working holiday makers are admitted to the UK on the condition that they do not have 'recourse to public funds'. In effect this means that for 12 months after they enter the country they cannot claim certain benefits that include: access to accommodation following homelessness, child benefit, disability living allowance, working tax credit, housing benefit, income support and other related allowances. EU Regulations do however enable workers and members of their families who move within the EU to take with them their acquired rights to social security and health care and careful advice should be taken on the rights of any migrant worker who becomes in need.

Learning point

For any migrant worker the acquisition of a National Insurance number must be a high priority as it not only legitimizes their position in the labour market but also, after some time in the country, enables them to access a range of state benefits and entitlements. Without access to a National Insurance number a migrant will find it impossible to open a bank account or a pension fund, or even work as a volunteer.

Given the complexity of the regulations and the insecure economic climate, issues surrounding access and eligibility for benefits and entitlements are often a source of problems and challenges for the migrant population as well as Gypsies and Travellers (who frequently share literacy issues with migrant workers; see further Chapter 11) and other vulnerable people. Particular problems relating to benefits include:

- difficulties in understanding the full range of benefits and entitlements available, eligibility criteria and procedures for accessing services and benefits;
- employers' lack of understanding and/or refusal to acknowledge a range of employees' rights in relation to work and related issues;
- procedural delays which can lead to destitution or loss of accommodation.

> ## Example
>
> Advice agencies report that workers often need help in completing forms for the Workers Registration Scheme[2] and to claim the benefits and tax credits to which they are legally entitled. Regulations and application forms can be very confusing for clients, particularly concerning change of circumstances for tax credits when moving between low-paid jobs.

Immigration issues

Given the range of work type and flexible opportunities for casual work available to migrants to rural areas, issues surrounding immigration status feature prominently in the concerns raised by workers. Although many of the reported issues surrounding immigration status appear to relate to 'undocumented' and 'illegal' workers, a number of situations and circumstances also present problems to those who have entered the country legitimately. In particular these relate to:

- problems with obtaining changes to work permits and associated difficulties in taking up another job;
- employment agencies providing incorrect information/advice about the immigration status of a worker;
- lack of clear concise explanations about what is required to legitimize their position from departments and agencies working with migrant workers.

Health

Significant anecdotal evidence existed to suggest that numerous health concerns were to be found among the migrant worker population in the area. However, prior to the research study being undertaken, little data existed to confirm these suspicions. Research findings established that there had not been a significant use of the health services by 'temporary' migrant workers in the years from the first waves of A8 migration until the study was undertaken. This was assumed to result from the fact that the majority of such workers were young men, a sector of the population that typically have a low level of health care needs. It was also assumed that workers were accessing services in other parts of the country when away from the Fenlands, or when returning to their country of origin on trips home.

However, the study identified a number of ongoing and unmet medical concerns, including stomach ulcers, asthma, heart and back problems and arthritis, some of which were exacerbated by working in fields or by packing house labour and/or living conditions. A number of cases of severe mental illness were found, similar to those noted among the Gypsy Traveller community when peer support and a change of environment occur, for example moving from a nomadic way of life to that of living in brick and mortar accommodation (Cemlyn et al. 2009). Gendered health differences were also noted, including migrant women reporting ongoing problems with sexual and reproductive health, including miscarriages (potentially exacerbated by undertaking heavy work) and the need to access terminations which can be problematic in terms of language barriers and access to NHS services.

Further work is currently ongoing to discover the extent to which mental health problems are either experienced or acknowledged within the migrant worker population. However, given the high degree of uncertainty, exploitation and fear in their lives, the level of isolation from any wider community, poor housing conditions and current dislocation, it would be reasonable to assume that there are ongoing and unrecognized mental health issues among many overseas workers (Carta et al. 2005).

Law and order and community cohesion

Issues such as crime, anti-social behaviour and access to policing and public safety services have been identified as significant issues affecting all local communities, migrant and indigenous alike. However, evidence was found of racist views and hostility in some areas which have experienced a large influx of migrants within a short time scale. In these localities far-right groups have gained adherents. Accordingly, a risk exists that migrant workers are vulnerable to hate crime. The overcrowded and physically insecure shared living conditions mean that migrant workers, and other vulnerable people living in such conditions (see further Chapter 6), are at risk of becoming victims of crimes such as theft and assault. For women in particular, there are risks of sexual assault within accommodation where shared bathroom and lavatory facilities exist. There is also evidence of alcohol-fuelled violence occurring between migrant workers, or conflicts over employment, which has on occasion led to serious assault and even murder. The knock-on effect of such incidents is increased fear (and potentially increased risk of racism) within the host community who have not been used to experiencing such problems in their neighbourhood (Clark 2007). Shamefully, some of the individuals involved in the worst exploitation of migrants have also been found to be involved in criminal activity, in some cases linked to sex trafficking and the drugs trade (Craig et al. 2007).

Example

Local Citizen Advice Bureaus (CABs) report that several clients have told staff that they have been made to sign their contracts of employment without having a chance to have these translated from English to their own language. Accordingly they do not know what they are signing or what their rights are. When some workers have asked for a copy of their contract, one gangmaster refused to let them have a copy, telling them that the Data Protection Act meant it could not be handed over.

Road safety

Road safety within Cambridgeshire by migrant drivers has posed an unprecedented problem, associated with the fact that in some cultures accepted driving practices within their home countries pose significant road safety risks when transposed to UK roads. Particular concern exists around attitudes to drink driving and seat belt usage. The Fenland Strategic Partnership has adopted the issue of migrant road users as a strategic theme and is working to improve road safety for everyone through developing a balanced 'education and enforcement' programme.

Community cohesion issues

Small incidents, such as tensions over resident parking spaces, collection of refuse, drinking in public open spaces, can all contribute to escalate public tensions and lead to a breakdown in community cohesion. Without therefore developing positive interactions between migrant communities and existing residents, it is impossible to take community cohesion and public safety for granted. Tensions between new and settled communities, whether this is Gypsy Travellers (formerly the largest minority ethnic community in Fenland) and/or A8 migrants and the indigenous communities, are often caused by a combination of myths and stereotypes and misinformation circulating and gaining currency. In the absence of any other information, media reporting can define local perceptions. Accordingly strategies for enhancing community cohesion need to involve a range of practical and attitudinal challenges to break down barriers to interaction.

Cross-cutting issues

In addition to the catalogue of specific issues identified, the problems facing vulnerable migrant workers are often exacerbated by the following factors which impact on every area of their lives:

- communications problems due to poor literacy or insufficient command of English;
- insufficient understanding of procedures, practices and legalities, for example motor insurance and employment registration.
- a culture of fear which often prevents a person from seeking assistance or help from 'outside' agencies, lest it results in loss of job, accommodation etc.[3]
- a work-dominated existence which curtails opportunities to develop social interaction with their local communities who themselves are sometimes cautious of or even hostile to any such interaction.

Migrant workers' sense of well-being and integration into the local population is therefore often negatively affected by a number of factors which exacerbate their vulnerability and can lead to increased risk of harm.

- Their precarious financial situation as a low-waged worker, together with worries about their inability to send remittances to their family by the time they have paid out for accommodation and other employer deductions.
- The yearning for contact with family members, but also the concern at their inability to adequately provide for family members who have travelled with them and who may have to live separately from the primary worker.
- Inadequate and expensive accommodation, which is sometimes unsafe and insecure.
- Difficulty in accessing English-language courses designed to meet their needs – often as a result of timing of classes or exhaustion after long hours of work

---

Example

An advice agency cites the case of a client who wants her boyfriend, who is the father of her child, to live with her. He is employed by a gangmaster who provides his accommodation in a shared house. The child's father has been told that if he leaves his accommodation to live with his girlfriend, he will be dismissed from his job. He will then be at risk of having to leave the country under the Workers' Registration Scheme.

Good practice in addressing migrant worker vulnerability

In Fenland in a pragmatic response to the issues already outlined, the local strategic partnership now acknowledged that migrant workers' issues need to be addressed by all partners in an integrated, holistic manner, which will improve individual vulnerabilities as well as enhance community cohesion in the locality.

A key strand in working with migrant workers consists of overcoming communication issues as the major challenge posed by the increasing number of migrant workers. Where language barriers exist, service providers face two particular problems:

- difficulties in understanding the true nature and extent of the problem(s) for which the client is seeking help, information, support or advice;
- difficulties in ensuring that the client fully understands the support available, or information and advice being given and its implications for his/her situation.

Translation service availability is a significant issue in the district as availability of translators is often poor, translation services can be expensive, or where volunteers are utilized, it can be difficult to obtain their services when required. While many voluntary and community projects are adopting innovative approaches to providing interpretation and translation (e.g by developing volunteers from Eastern Europe to help in community translations and pre-ESOL training with their own community so that migrant workers gain a basic understanding of English and can make themselves better understood), the growing cultural and linguistic diversity of the migrant labour force means that this issue remains a major challenge.

Learning point

All agencies which come into contact with migrant workers should take responsibility for issues relating to their needs, rather than constantly seeking to refer the issue and individual to another organization which is seen as 'expert' in working with migrants.

Actions to support potentially vulnerable migrant workers must encompass tackling discrimination and racism, while enabling them to have access to information and advice, access to health, housing and other public services

> alongside advice and support to obtain employment or to set up in business as a self-employed person.

Agencies in Fenland are being actively encouraged to work alongside the Employment Tribunal system (including ACAS – the body which can provide conciliation in employment disputes) and in partnership with the Small Business Service, the Health and Safety Executive, the Gang Master Licensing Authority, the Commission for Equality and Human Rights and other governmental agencies who have contact with migrant workers. The main aim of the strategy is to ensure a joined-up approach to delivering advice, guidance and practical business support for small employers, as well as a proactive (but educational rather than punitive) approach to compliance and, where necessary, legal enforcement to ensure protection of vulnerable migrant workers.

A further strand of the strategy has involved the development of a Diverse Community Forum, initiated by Fenland District Council and partner agencies. This consists of a network of statutory, community and voluntary organizations who are committed to addressing vulnerability among migrant worker populations and promoting equality of opportunities, social justice, good community relations, and respect for human rights.

To meet the planned objectives referred to above, the Fora has undertaken the following actions:

- produced a booklet and online website for migrant workers providing information about services in Fenland;
- produced a DVD and oral/spoken 'New Arrivals Pack' to support vulnerable new migrants and others who require information in these formats;
- provided 'drop-in' centres at community hubs to provide practical advice and information;
- provided kiosks in community centres which link advice seekers to professional advisors;
- provided 'Migrant Population Advisors' in Council one-stop-shops thus enabling people to access information from advisors of their own cultural/linguistic background;
- employed Eastern European Police Community Support Officers to engage with migrants around crime and safety issues;
- produced a joint strategic health needs assessment;
- provided a hostel for those without recourse to public funds to enable accommodation in emergency situations and to address homelessness and the vulnerability issues which arise from such status.

Learning point

How do these activities help vulnerable migrant workers in the local community?

- By drawing together a wide range of information into accessible locations and providing expertise and understanding of the needs of migrant workers in a non-threatening environment.
- By providing space for developing dialogue, trust and working relations between and within organizations, the migrant worker communities and the wider population.
- By strengthening the contribution of the third sector to community cohesion and development by enabling them to share their expertise.
- By holding regular meetings to bring together Fora members to share information and develop good practice in service provision and delivery.
- By enabling the Fora to commission research and run seminars across the locality to advance knowledge and increase understanding between different sectors of the community.
- By bringing people together in partnership to work with and support vulnerable migrant workers.

Conclusion

This case study emphasizes the difficulties which can face both migrant workers and the wider host community at times of transition. In Fenland we recognize that if conditions are not actively created which support the integration of migrant workers and their families, the seeds are sown for vulnerability, social exclusion and segregation. By failing to recognize and actively support cultural diversity, racism and xenophobia are reinforced and given a dangerous legitimacy. Many European countries with a history of inward migration are now struggling with these issues due to their failure to develop or implement inclusive integration strategies from an early stage of the migration process.

The conditions under which people can enter and reside in a country have significant consequences for most areas of public policy, including labour rights, political participation, social protection, education and training. If immigration policy is designed to keep migrant workers and their families in the status of temporary mobile workers, the likely result is that settlement will take place under ethically unsatisfactory and discriminatory conditions leading to situations which can potentially place vulnerable workers at great (and preventable) risk of harm.

Within this chapter it is therefore stressed that to enhance community cohesion and safeguard vulnerable adults, both front line staff and wider consortiums of service providers need to focus on developing initiatives that forge links between the settled community and new arrivals, for example mentoring programmes, and maximizing opportunities for people to mix, socialize and celebrate the diversity of the area. In developing strategies for integration, cohesion and to protect vulnerable migrant workers it is also recommended that information and training materials emphasize both the migrant population's significant contribution to the (rural) economy and also that they are often victims of exploitation and discrimination by both their employers and the wider community, leading to isolation, and a popular public emphasis on community differences rather than similarities and shared rights.

When developing schemes and initiatives, however, it is particularly important to recognize that the migrant workforce is not a static body and that its composition changes depending on migration flows in and out of the UK, thus, a migrant workforce that might be identified as consisting of a particular national group in one year may be made up of a different group the following year. In order to ensure that we are meeting needs in a responsive manner, the Fenland local strategic partnership reviews the evidence and key issues on an annual basis and considers the case for adjustments in policies, procedures and practices to ensure all services meet the needs of our evolving community. We would recommend that this practice is followed in any locality seeking to engage with vulnerable migrant populations.

Notes

1   The Gangmasters (Licensing) Act 2004 (c.11) was passed in response to the deaths of 21 Chinese shellfish collectors 'Cocklers' who were made to work in dangerous circumstances by the agency who had brought them to the UK for work-related purposes. The Act, which regulates and licenses 'gangmasters' and monitors the circumstances and conditions of vulnerable workers in agricultural work, shellfish collecting and related packing industries defines a 'gangmaster' as someone who 'supplies a worker' to undertake employment in the industries listed above.

2   Under the Workers' Registration Scheme all new A8 migrant workers coming to Britain for employment purposes have to register for the first 12 months after they enter the UK to allow monitoring of their employment activities (www.ukba.homeoffice.gov.uk/workingintheuk/eea/wrs/).

3   The right to work/reside regime under the Workers Registration Scheme has, to a large extent, exacerbated this problem due to the requirement that migrant workers must not have a break of employment exceeding 30 days during the first 12 months of residence in the UK.

References

Carta, M., Bernal, M., Hardoy, M. and Haro-Abad, J.-M. (2005) Migration and mental health in Europe. *Clinical Practice and Epidemiology in Mental Health*, 13: 1–13.

Cemlyn, S., Greenfields, M., Burnett, S., Matthews, Z. and Whitwell, C. (2009) *Review of Inequalities Experienced by Gypsy and Traveller Communities*. London. Equalities and Human Rights Commission (EHRC).

Clark, R. (2007) The great British migration scandal. *The Times*, 20 September.

Craig, G., Gaus, A., Wilkinson, M., Skrivankova, K. and McQuade, A. (2007) *Modern Slavery in the United Kingdom*. York: Joseph Rowntree Foundation.

Department for Work and Pensions (DWP) (2006), *The Impact of Free Movement of Workers from Central and Eastern Europe on the UK Labour Market*. Working Paper No. 29. London: DWP.

Glossop, C. and Shaheen, F. (2009) *Accession to Recession: A8 Migration in Bristol and Hull*. London: Centre for Cities.

International Labour Organization (2009) *Protecting the Rights of Migrant Workers: A Shared Responsibility*. Geneva: International Labour Office.

Jayaweera, H. and Anderson, B. (2009) *Migrant Workers and Vulnerable Employment: A Review of Existing Data – A Report for the TUC Commission on Vulnerable Employment*. London: Centre on Migration, Policy and Society.

McKay, S. and Winkelmann-Gleed, A. (2005) *Migrant Workers in the East of England*. Cambridge: EEDA.

Milmo, C. (2007) Isolated, intimidated and undermined: the immigrants building a new life in the Fens. *Independent*, 22 September.

Robinson, V. (2002) *Migrant Workers in the UK*. London: Department of Work and Pensions.

Scottish Association of Citizens Advice Bureaux (SACAB) *Migrant Workers Are Finding Scotland Hard Work, Says CAB Service*. Press Release, available at: www.cas.org.uk/pressrelease1262006.aspx.

Winder, R. (2005) *Bloody Foreigners: The History of Immigration to Britain*. London: Abacus.

Further resources

Concordia (2006) *Migrant Workers in Northern Ireland: Meeting the Needs of Migrant Workers, Their Families and Their Employers*. Dungannon: Concordia.

Dench, S., Hurstfield, J., Hill, D. and Ackroyd, K. (2006) *Employers' Use of Migrant Labour Summary Report*. London: Home Office. Available at: http://rds.homeoffice.gov.uk/rds/pdfs06/rdsolr0306.pdf

ECCR (2009) *Vulnerable Migrant Workers: The Responsibility of Business*. Oxford: ECCR.

Kofman, E., Lukes, S., D'Angelo, A. and Montagna, N. (2009) *The Equality Implications of Being a Migrant in Britain*. Manchester: Equality and Human Rights Commission.

Welsh Local Government Association webpage: *Migrant Workers in Wales* (includes statistics and links to publications), www.wlga.gov.uk/english/migrant-workers-in-wales/

13 Conclusion

Margaret Greenfields, Roger Dalrymple and Agnes Fanning

The array of chapters and case studies assembled in this book provide theoretical and practical insight into a range of vulnerabilities and risk factors, encountered at different life-stages and in different domains of health, well-being and socio-economic disadvantage. While predominantly focusing their chapter around a single characteristic or circumstance of risk, each author also notes the cumulative impacts of intersectional disadvantage (Collins 2000) which may exacerbate powerlessness and lessen the opportunities for individuals within these situations to engage with services. From a theorized perspective, these examples reflect Gidden's (1991) 'narrative of the self' as ontological security is situated in a state of heightened risk when an inability exists to effectively challenge the myriad buffets of a threatening world.

While at first sight many of the vulnerabilities considered within this collection are identity-based and associated with particular groups of individuals whose susceptibility to risk is sometimes innate, sometimes acquired but sufficiently distinctive that they can be identified as discrete groups in popular imagination, political rhetoric and legislation, it rapidly becomes clear that each chapter in this book has sought to move beyond an identity-based conceptualization of what it means to be 'at risk' or vulnerable in modern western societies. Indeed, a cumulative theme emerging from the preceding chapters is the notion that identity-based accounts of vulnerability and risk are inadequate to convey the dynamic and unpredictable process by which sudden change (and ultimately disadvantage) may be visited upon any citizen at any time, an awareness elegantly captured by Bauman (2000) in his contemplation of 'liquid modernity'. Indeed Bauman's (1989) exposition of the reactive phenomenon of heterophobia ('resentment of the different') holds relevance for understanding the barriers to social inclusion and discriminatory treatment experienced by many of those who are the subject of chapters within this text, especially those who are frequently positioned in normative discourse as responsible for their own plight through mal-location by virtue of ethnicity; socio-economic status or moral reprehensibility (e.g. migrant workers, prisoners, the homeless) or who (like Gypsies and Travellers or the mentally ill) are the subject of socially constructed moral panics (Goode and Ben-Yahuda 1994). In contrast, the categorization of older people, and those with physical or intellectual impairments (for example) as innately 'at risk', while reflecting the stark reality that certain groups and individuals are significantly more vulnerable to harm and exploitation than are others, fails often to reflect the richness of experience, desire for autonomy and self-knowledge which exists among members of these (often under-valued) groups within society. Accordingly, within this book authors have sought to provide a more nuanced understanding of the lived realities of people who are all too frequently marginalized and silenced, allowing the reader to contemplate both societal and structural neglect of certain individuals and their *own* reflexive response to those groups included herein. While the design of the current book aims to facilitate browsing and consultation of relevant chapters out of sequence according to readers' interests and professional preoccupations, this short conclusion will seek to draw out four dominant themes and concerns from the book as a whole. These are first that policymakers and practitioners do well to understand and approach vulnerability and risk holistically in recognition of the intersections of risk and the dynamic nature of vulnerability (see further Alwang et al. 2001) explored in the preceding chapters. Second, we suggest that there is considerable benefit in approaching our work with at-risk adults relationally, retaining a clear sense of the embedded nature of vulnerable adults in wider social networks and recognizing that some dimensions of the disadvantage they face derives from social perceptions and attitudes (Oliver and Sapey 2006; Bennett et al. 2009) an approach explicitly recognized in British policy terms with the advent of the Equality Act 2010, albeit the legislation as enacted regrettably fails to implement (anticipated) duties on public bodies with regard to socio-economic status as a cause of inequality. Third, we suggest the value, especially for new and developing practitioners, of understanding risk and vulnerability discursively, recognizing the extent to which concepts of vulnerability and disadvantage are variously defined across cultures and political hegemonies (Potter 1996). Finally, we follow an emerging body of theory and practice in arguing the critical importance of understanding 'at risk' adults subjectively, constructing them not as 'other' but, wherever possible, putting ourselves in their shoes, and recognizing our common vulnerabilities (Leonard 1997; Martin and Knox 2000; Thompson and Thompson 2001; Burke and Harrison 2002). By engaging with these humanistic (and, we suggest, ethical) approaches to working with adults 'at risk of harm' the reflexive practitioner obtains a comprehension of the particular challenges experienced by individuals from vulnerable groups or at intersectional points in their life-course, enabling a rich inter-disciplinary overview to be taken, while deepening awareness of one's own professional practice.

Understanding risk and vulnerability holistically

The dynamic and changing nature of risk and vulnerability are patent from the preceding chapters. The dyad of chapters dealing with the lifespan from early adulthood to older age (Potter and Fanning) highlight and comment upon these crucial junctures in life (young parenthood and ageing) which can so easily open onto vulnerability and disadvantage. That vulnerability is often intergenerational will be apparent from the many overlaps and cross-references within these contributions. The companion chapters by Burton, Parris, Mgutshini, Farquharson and Aitken, Cole and Greenfields demonstrate those domains of vulnerability in which individuals may, by contrast, find themselves at any stage of the life-cycle. The case studies and vignettes supplied in each chapter give plentiful illustration of how different domains of vulnerability may overlap, deepening exclusion and increasing the 'hard-to-reach' nature of many vulnerable individuals. Indeed, it is not uncommon that the substance user and the insecurely accommodated young parent with mental health challenges transpire to be one and the same person.

Considerable evidence exists in relation to the long-term and often intergenerational impacts of exclusion and vulnerability on health, education and life-chance outcomes (Davey-Smith 2003; Feinstein and Sabates 2006), although less is known about the impacts of multiple and intersectional risks experienced by marginalized individuals and groups across the 'protected characteristics' outlined within the Equalities Act 2010 (specifically race and ethnicity, gender, disability, age, sexual orientation, faith and belief, transgender status, marriage/civil partnership and maternity status). The Equality and Human Rights Commission's (EHRC) first trienniel review, *How Fair Is Britain* (2010), brought together evidence from a range of sources, including Census data, surveys and research, to expose the ways in which life for certain groups or people with specific characteristics failed starkly to match up to the ideals of equality expounded upon in policy statements and enshrined within the Equality Act. The acknowledged limitations on knowledge in relation to some of those most vulnerable people, not least the lack of nuance in relation to age-gender-race-disability intersectionality and the ways in which these different characteristics can segue into a situation of multiple and deep exclusion are outlined in considerable depth within that report, which cautions against complacence in relation to apparent advances in equality.

The evidential weight of numerous reports and research findings in relation to vulnerability by characteristics all argue for the need to conceive of at-risk groups in as holistic a manner as possible. While policy initiatives and support packages must by need adopt labels and descriptors in designing and delivering social protection interventions, it is self-evident that individual practitioners should remain mindful of the inter-connectedness of different groups and the systemic nature of disadvantage and deprivation in 21st-century Britain.

Initiatives to embody this holistic approach in 'joined up' organization and policymaking were initially developed in 1997 under the auspices of the then incoming Labour administration with the formation of a Government Social Exclusion Unit (subsequently the Social Exclusion Task Force until it was abolished in November 2010 and the functions of the Task Force subsumed into the Coalition Government's Office of Civil Society), which was tasked with delivering a range of services to the most disadvantaged members of society, including groups and individuals identified within the chapters in this volume. The broad sweep of the Social Exclusion Unit included government recognition of the impacts of financial, and economic insecurity, stigma, disability and frequent movement upon individuals who were already vulnerable, or who were potentially 'at risk' as a result of such stressors. While the political landscape within which such policies and the Social Inclusion Unit were created has disappeared, perhaps never to return, the innovation of the vision of 'community' and 'civil society' has become embedded into political rhetoric and forms the cornerstone of the present government's 'Big Society' agenda, albeit with the intent that individuals, communities and voluntary sector agencies will undertake the activities which were formerly within the purview of the State (Peck 2010). This transfer of responsibilities from the State to knowledgeable voluntary sector agencies and the notion of an active civil society where communities develop cohesive policies and care for their members themselves, is not without adherents, with the National Council for Voluntary Organizations (the umbrella body for third-sector agencies formed in 1919) having delivered a manifesto on this topic in 2009.

In a large part, such determination for communities and individuals to wrest control of assets from the state, and free up activities can be argued to stem from a reaction to excessive 'governmentality' (the concept pertaining to the control techniques by which Governments render citizens 'governable' coined by Foucault and explored in depth by Dean 1999). In the latter days of the New Labour administration, policymaking designing to counter the dynamic and unpredictable nature of risk became somewhat heavy-handed and inflexible. Laudable initiatives to protect a range of vulnerable groups including the homeless, people with disabilities or children, and a consciously 'risk-averse' administration engaged in a project to protect citizens against a world, perceived of as dangerous and hostile, resulted in a raft of 'restrictive regulation and tighter regulatory controls aimed at securing the self regulation of welfare providers and welfare recipients alike' (May et al. 2005: 4). During this era not only restrictive policing policies but also 'safeguarding' legislation, much of it produced in response to high-profile instances of neglect and harm (see further Cole at Chapter 7 on the control demonization of prisoners) grew exponentially. Blanket measures designed to guard against escalation of risk became applied to those working with a whole range of vulnerable individuals and safeguarding policymaking initiatives had gathered such momentum by the end of the Labour term of office that civil liberties concerns were increasingly raised (and not only by opposition parties) about the extent to which the State's concern to safeguard and protect was in fact impinging upon individual freedoms (Savage 2009). Objections to the 'vetting and barring' register, the proposed system of identity cards, and the ever-increasing require-ment for criminal-records checking even for individuals involved in the most cursory contact with vulnerable groups led to accusations that initially well-intentioned initiatives had given way to a 'nanny state' and to intolerable levels of surveillance and scrutiny of the citizenry. This momentum towards increased state involvement in safeguarding has been dramatically arrested with the formation of the coalition administration in May 2010 whose cross-party membership coalesced strongly around notions of increased civil liber-ties and the need to roll back an overly intrusive state. Eighteen months into the new administration (at the time of going to press) the former administra-tion's planned programme for the issuance of identity cards has been discon-tinued and criminal record checks and vetting and barring regimes have been scaled back significantly, with the explicit intent of restoring civil liberties and enabling greater access to volunteering opportunities for those who wish to participate in the 'Big Society' project through supporting potentially 'at risk' groups.

While at the time of going to press, the engagement between state, civil society and (explicitly) the voluntary and third sector remains in a state of flux, with regard to respective roles in deliverance of services to vulnerable and 'at risk' individuals and groups, it is inevitable that as the 'Big Society' model becomes established a more holistic approach to comprehension of risk will occur, as front line practitioners are (as demonstrated within this book) often significantly better placed than policymakers working within a leviathan system to understand the myriad strands which impact and resonate in the lives of service users.

Understanding risk and vulnerability relationally

A second core theme arising from the preceding chapters in this volume is the value of understanding risk and vulnerability not in isolation for particular groups or individuals, but relationally to the wider networks and frames of refer-ence supplied by society. A number of the chapters allude to Maslow's (1943) influential 'hierarchy of needs' as a conceptual framework for understanding disadvantage and deprivation in society. In Maslow's terms, the at-risk or vulnerable adult is denied 'self actualization' – full realization of individual aptitudes, aspirations and potentialities – by frustration of their lower order needs (e.g. accommodation, adequate diet and the meeting of other physiological needs) resulting from physical or mental impairment, socioeconomic disadvantage or other circumstances. In considering how best policymakers and practitioners can design interventions and ameliorations for this constituency, Maslow's theory can helpfully be brought into dialogue with Axel Honneth's (1996) work on the relations of power, recognition and respect. Marrying these two elements enables us to contemplate *relational* thinking about vulnerability and empowerment. Honneth argues that disadvantaged and deprived social roles are not the result of fixed and immutable characteristics of the disadvantaged groups in question but are the result of social definition and lack of recognition of the potential value to society of such groups. As his translator, Joel Anderson, notes in the introduction to a seminal Honneth text:

> Regularly, members of marginalized and subaltern groups have been systematically denied recognition for the worth of their culture or way of life, the dignity of their status as persons, and the inviolability of their physical integrity.
>
> (Honneth 1996: x)

Honneth's approach is valuable in helping us to realize that vulnerable and at-risk identities are to some extent created *relationally*, hence social definitions, and the ascription or withdrawal of social capital to individuals make a crucial difference to their position in society. By constructing individuals or groups as defined by an *absence* of higher level functioning or lack of self-actualization and utilizing this deficiency model to focus on their non-normative or socially challenging status such members of society are diminished and located within marginal categories which emphasize their 'difference' from whom *we* are or to the status to which we aspire.

Foucault's (1963) discourse on the medicalization of sexuality and mental illness and 'the gaze' of medical scrutiny which characterizes certain behaviours as in need of 'treatment' and 'cure' epitomizes the high point of such constitutions of pathologized 'difference'. While in the early 21st century (as explored within Harries' and Mgutshini's chapters) attitudes towards sexual orientation and mental illness are perceived of very differently from in the past, when they were routinely regarded as abnormal conditions requiring punishment, long-term hospitalization or 'treatment', tragically a sense of fear and prejudice still prevails among some individuals and in some communities, exposing lesbian, gay, bi-sexual and transgender people, and those individuals with mental health conditions to ridicule, stigma and hatred.

While changing terms and characterizations of the 'despised other' vary across time and place, so that (contemporaneously) poverty and lack of educational attainment are (in many social circles, and indeed in the sense of policy and legal preoccupations) regarded as more discreditable than are obvious physical disability or learning impairment, the social construction of what is, and is not, 'socially acceptable', and thus, that which is thus 'abnormal' and seen as constituting a social 'risk', varies within cultural groupings, and across age bands. Accordingly for some sectors of society, a vacuous 'celebrity culture' predicated on physical attractiveness or closely prescribed corporeal capitals, may be perceived of as something to be aspired to, and in contrast an elderly or physically disabled person with a fascinating history and wealth of experience may be subject to abuse and hate crime (EHRC 2009) and ridiculed as being 'useless'. While it is tempting to consider that the advent of such legislation as the Equality Act 2010 equates to a universal recognition of the value of all people, and particularly those with protected characteristics, the evidence which demonstrates the stark variability of treatment of discrete groups, and the discussions within the chapters in this book which explore the numerous ways in which 'risk' can exist, remain a pertinent reminder of the relational domains of vulnerability.

Understanding risk and vulnerability discursively

To develop the previous point in greater depth, there is obvious value for astute and developing practitioners in understanding risk and vulnerability discursively, that is, in remaining alert to the ways in which different discourses characterize and sometimes stigmatize different groups as being at risk at different times in history and across the life-course. Similarly, the social protection measures designed by varying administrations take on their own character and make use of their own discourses to frame discussions of vulnerability. Where, for example, a 2009 discussion of the topic of 'risk' would have centred upon the then Government's favoured terms of 'safeguarding' and 'vulnerable adults' (see further Fairclough 2000 and Worley 2005 for a discussion on 'language slippage'), it is already apparent that the coalition administration is evolving a differently nuanced discourse to address these themes within the context of the 'Big Society'. The shift towards volunteerism and the roll-back of the state which is underway at the time of going to press deliberately encourages a decline in risk-laden terminology, and hand-in-hand with the opening of opportunities for third-sector agencies to build upon their knowledge base and deliver services, an increase in positivist approaches which will ultimately rely on evidence-based findings (and the inevitable human cost of such errors) before acknowledging that certain individuals are at greater risk and that state intervention may be required to improve their life-chances and minimize characteristic-based vulnerabilities.

The book's chapters, alert to the changing climate of service delivery, thus constitute not a series of portraits of 'at-risk' adults in modern society but rather a collage or palimpsest, each permutation of vulnerability and risk over-lapping with and growing out of the last to create a series of augmented reali-ties. This collage is presented not as a deterministic model – where one form of vulnerability must *inevitably* open onto the next – but in an attempt to encourage holistic practice and informed interventions which are cognisant of the established connections between different forms of disadvantage and exclusion, and which, it is to be hoped, can act as 'short circuits' to ameliorate the harm experienced by an individual free-falling into risk.

Understanding risk and vulnerability subjectively

The final theme which we present within this text relates to the recognition of the proliferating risks and vulnerabilities within the post-modern world. Beck's (1992) conceptualization of the 'risk society' has gained currency since the terrorist outrages of 9/11 (and subsequent international conflagrations and natural disasters) have served to compound fears in the popular consciousness of sudden catastrophe and misfortune. As noted earlier, an increased recogni-tion that 'we are all vulnerable now' has pervasively informed policy and prac-tice interventions across the western world in the past decade – ranging from heightened security measures in public locations (Liberty 2003, 2007), to substantial 'health and safety' interventions which have been identified as limiting children's opportunities for creative and healthy play (Gleave 2008) and overwhelmingly, in the early years of the 21st century, permeated legisla-tion aimed at supporting potentially at-risk children and adults. In a thought-provoking article, Fineman (2008) goes so far as to theorize the vulnerable subject as the most apposite model for negotiating the balance between indi-vidual freedom and the State. Rather than, as currently, placing the autono-mous, Lockean, liberal citizen (Locke 1977) at the core of all social and legislative discourse, Fineman argues that we would do better to give primacy to the vulnerable subject in all such contexts:

> Far more representative of actual lived experience and the human condition, the vulnerable subject should be at the center of our polit-ical and theoretical endeavors. The vision of the state that would emerge in such an engagement would be more responsive to and responsible for the vulnerable subject.
>
> (2008: 2)

Fineman's approach harmonizes with the proposition emerging both from each of the preceding chapters and the above discussion on comprehension of 'risk status' that identity-based accounts of vulnerability fail to acknowledge first how one vulnerability can so easily open onto another and second, how any individual, at any point in the lifespan, can readily fall prey to vulnerability, find themselves classified as 'at risk' and in need of support and re-empowerment, which may or may not (depending upon how the risk status is perceived and the degree of 'innocence' or blame attached to the status) be forthcoming. Thus the discrete chapters included in this volume may provide a window onto others' vulnerability but they equally hold a mirror up to society's own appropriation of vulnerability and fears for the future. We therefore invite the critical reader to contemplate their own subjective consideration of the nature of risk and risk-aversion and how individual behaviour patterns (and expectations) may intersect with our willingness to engage with the often difficult topics considered within these pages.

Conclusion

While the increased recognition of intersectionality of risk has translated (with in some cases great effectiveness) into third-sector and state structures of support, care and 're-empowerment' (Fineman 2008) the grounds of legal action of the basis of multiple forms of discrimination remains (at the time of going to press) outside of the implemented terms of the Equality Act 2010. The explanation cited for this situation is the complicated and cumbersome nature of legal action for multiple and intersectional discrimination. If policymakers and legal experts consider such porous and permeable grounds of exclusion and discrimination unduly complex, then, for front-line practitioners and service users, therefore, while certain situations reveal heightened risk, deeper vulnerability and more negative outcomes, the challenges of retaining a truly holistic perspective in practice remain considerable. More than one of the preceding chapters cites the recent high-profile cases in adult and children's social care where insufficient 'joined-up' working among health and social care professionals contributed to vulnerable individuals falling through the net of care provision. While the findings of subsequent inquiries and reviews brought censure and in some cases dismissal of individual practitioners, the failures in these instances in part reflect the considerable challenge of integrating all the constituencies involved in health and social care provision to the extent that their interactions with each area of disadvantage, exclusion and vulnerability add up to a coherent picture where risks can be identified and appropriate interventions made.

The past 40 years have seen very significant progress in terms of recognition and protection for at-risk adults in society. Disadvantaged groups who would have been effectively hidden from public notice a matter of decades ago are now increasingly the focus of ameliorative and reformist social policy. Yet further progress is needed if the empowerment of excluded and vulnerable people is to be realized with true equity across the regions of the United

Kingdom. Practice, policy and fiscal responses indeed vary across the constituent nations of Britain with Scotland in particular being at the forefront of well-resourced, imaginative and social progressive policies, such as those which seek to eliminate homelessness within a few short years (see Greenfields' chapter).

The majority of inequalities and vulnerabilities we explore within this book do, however, relate to economic exclusion. As is clear from many of the foregoing chapters, access to financial security is in many ways the single most protective factor for any vulnerable individual or group regardless of age, physical or mental impairment. With access to money, personalized, individual, high-quality services and support can be purchased to support individuals who would otherwise be at risk of harm. The Marmot Review (2010) noted that access to higher education and resultant increased income levels accorded with a significant reduction in premature death. While we do not claim that education, employment and higher income are a universal panacea for adults who are at risk of harm, we regret that the implementation of the Equality Act 2010 has not included the intended clause which placed a duty on public bodies to take account of the socio-economic status of local constituents and service users. We would argue that even as a symbolic act such implementation would have highlighted the understanding that income inequalities enhance vulnerability and risk across the life-course. At this time of fundamental change in British social policy and practice, we can merely offer this text as a small contribution to broadening understanding in the hope that for some at-risk adults at least, the effective and informed work of committed practitioners can lead to a reduction in vulnerability, disadvantage and actual harm.

References

Alwang, J., Siegel, P. and Jørgensen, S. (2001) *Vulnerability: A View From Different Disciplines*. Washington, DC: Social Protection Unit, The World Bank.

Bauman, Z. (1989) *Modernity and the Holocaust*. Cambridge: Polity.

Bauman, Z. (2000) *Liquid Modernity*. Cambridge: Polity.

Beck, U. (1992) *The Risk Society: Towards A New Modernity*. London: Sage.

Bennett, T., Savage, M., Silva, E., Warde, A., Gayo-Cal, M. and Wright, D. (2009) *Culture, Class, Distinction*. London: Routledge.

Burke, B. and Harrison, P. (2002) Anti-oppressive practice. In R. Adams, L. Dominelli and M. Payne (eds) *Anti-oppressive Practice*. Basingstoke: Palgrave Macmillan.

Collins, P. (2000) *Black Feminist Thought: Knowledge, Consciousness, and the Politics of Empowerment*. New York: Routledge.

Davey-Smith, G. (ed.) (2003) *Health Inequalities: Life Course Approaches (Studies in Poverty, Inequality & Social Exclusion)*. Bristol: Policy.

Dean, M. (1999) *Governmentality: Power and Rule in Modern Society*. London: Sage.

Equality and Human Rights Commission (EHRC) (2009) *Promoting the Safety and Security of Disabled People*. London: EHRC.

Equality and Human Rights Commission (EHRC) (2010) *First Triennial Review: How Fair Is Britain?* London: EHRC.

Fairclough, N. (2000) *New Labour: New Language?* London: Routledge.

Feinstein, L. and Sabates, R. (2006) *Predicting Adult Life Outcomes from Earlier Signals: Identifying Those at Risk*. London: The Cabinet Office.

Fineman, M.A. (2008) The vulnerable subject: anchoring equality in the human condition. *Yale Journal of Law and Feminism*, 20(1): 1–23.

Foucault, F. (1963) *The Birth of the Clinic: An Archaeology of Medical Perception*. New York: Vintage.

Giddens, A. (1991) *Modernity and Self-identity: Self and Society in the Late Modern Age*. Cambridge: Polity.

Gleave, J. (2008) *Risk and Play: A Literature Review*. London: PlayDay.

Goode, E. and Ben Yehuda, N. (1994) *Moral Panics: The Social Construction of Deviance*. Oxford: Blackwell.

Honneth, A. (1996) *The Struggle for Recognition: The Moral Grammar of Social Conflicts*. Cambridge: Polity.

Leonard, P. (1997) *Post-modern Welfare: Reconstructing an Emancipatory Project*. Thousand Oaks, CA: Sage.

Liberty (2003) *Casualty of War Counter-terror Legislation in Rural England*. London: NCCL.

Liberty (2007) *Overlooked: Surveillance and Personal Privacy in Modern Britain*. London: NCCL.

Locke, J. (1977) *Two Treatises of Government*. London: Dent Everyman's Library.

Marmot Review (2010) *Fair Society: Healthy Lives – Strategic Review of Health Inequalities in England Post 2010*. Available at: www.marmot-review.org.uk/.

Martin, J. and Knox, J. (2000) Methodological and ethical issues in research on lesbians and gay men. *Social Work Research*, 24: 51–9.

Maslow, A. (1943) A theory of human motivation. *Psychological Review*, 50(4): 370–96.

May, J., Cloke, P. and Johnsen, S. (2005) Re-phasing neoliberalism: New Labour and Britain's crisis of street homelessness. *Antipode*, 37(4): 703–30.

National Council for Voluntary Organizations (NCVO) (2009) *Civil Society: A Framework for Action*. London: NCVO.

Oliver, M. and Sapey, B. (2006) *Social Work with Disabled People*. Basingstoke: Palgrave Macmillan.

Peck, J. (2010) *Big Society: Small State*. Available at: www.respublica.org.uk/blog/2010/08/big-society-small-state#comments.

Potter, J. (1996) *Representing Reality: Discourse, Rhetoric and Social Construction*. London: Sage.

Savage, M. (2009) Revealed: the full extent of Labour's curbs on civil liberties: Audit report highlights 'permanent erosion' of freedoms since 1997. *Independent*, 20 February.

Thompson, N. and Thompson, S. (2001) Empowering older people: beyond the care model. *Journal of Social Work*, 1(1): 61–76.

Williams, M. (2005) Tolerable liberalism. In A. Eisenberg and J. Spinner-Halev (eds) *Minorities Within Minorities*. Cambridge: Cambridge University Press.

Worley, C. (2005) 'It's not about race. It's about the community': New Labour and 'community cohesion'. *Critical Social Policy*, 25(4): 483–96.

Index

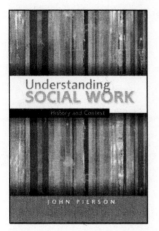

UNDERSTANDING SOCIAL WORK

John Pierson

9780335237951 (Paperback)
2011

eBook also available

The evolution of social work across the twentieth century offers a rich source of insight and inspiration for contemporary practice. It is essential that students new to social work understand how it has been shaped by past events and what this means for the future of social work and their roles as social workers.

This volume draws on archival material, social policy, normative theory and human rights doctrines to dissolve the border between past and present. Focused specifically on the UK, each chapter explains concisely how current practice was shaped by, and developed from efforts to build the 'decent society'.

Key features:

- Written in an accessible style and format that stimulates discussion
- Features case studies demonstrating specific approaches and styles of decision-making
- Contains exercises and extracts from the writings of prominent experts

www.openup.co.uk

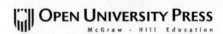
OPEN UNIVERSITY PRESS
McGraw · Hill Education